The Physical Principles of
Computed Tomography

THE LITTLE, BROWN LIBRARY OF RADIOLOGY
Herbert L. Abrams, M.D., Series Editor

The Physical Principles of Computed Tomography

William R. Hendee, Ph.D.

Professor and Chairman
Department of Radiology
University of Colorado Health Sciences Center
Denver, Colorado

LITTLE, BROWN AND COMPANY, BOSTON/TORONTO

TO THE MEMORY OF MARVIN M. D. WILLIAMS, PH.D.,
AN INSPIRATION FOR ALL THOSE WHO FOLLOW
IN MEDICAL PHYSICS

Contents

Preface

In the early 1970s, x-ray transmission computed tomography entered the medical arena and initiated a series of developments that are now recognized as a revolution in diagnostic imaging. For the first time, computers were inserted between the process of accumulating radiologic data about the patient and that of producing the final images for interpretation by the physician. This introduction of the computer and mathematical algorithms for data manipulation into the field of diagnostic imaging has led to increased reliance on quality assurance measures to ensure that images furnished by computed tomographic units depict pathology present in the patient rather than artifacts arising in the image-forming process. The presence of the computer and the complex methods of processing x-ray transmission data also have increased the demand on physicists and engineers to monitor the imaging process to prevent misinterpretation of the resulting pictures. Finally, the advent of computed tomography introduced the use of digital techniques for data processing in diagnostic imaging, and this approach is now developing rapidly in more conventional areas of radiology such as roentgenography and ultrasound as well as in emerging modalities including positron tomography and nuclear magnetic-resonance imaging.

Computed tomography has affected diagnostic imaging in other ways. For example, the exquisite rendition of low-contrast information in x-ray transmission computed tomography has produced a growing awareness of the importance of low-contrast perceptibility in other imaging modalities. This awareness has led to the identification of methods to enhance contrast resolution in other modalities, and the development and clinical application of these methods have become prime areas for research. The apparent high expense of computed tomography as an imaging process certainly has not escaped the attention of government officials concerned with the increasing cost of health care. In many communities, requests for acquisition of computed tomographic units have blazed the trail through the legal processes associated with certificate-of-need legislation and the establishment of health systems agencies.

The interface between x-ray transmission computed tomography and the physician employing the technique for patient diagnosis is a complex one requiring at least a moderate level of knowledge about the equipment on the part of the physician. In addition, an in-depth understanding of the equipment and of approaches to data processing is essential for the physicist or engineer responsible for the proper operation of the computed tomographic unit. Technologists using a computed tomographic unit need to be familiar with at least the rudiments of the computed tomographic process. It is for all these professionals that this text is written.

For physicians involved in the interface between computed tomography and patient diagnosis, the text is intended to convey a reasonable amount of information about the principles of computed tomography. For physicists and engineers interested in computed tomography, the text is intended as an introduction to the discipline. Technologists working in computed tomography may wish to pick and choose topics in the book, depending on their needs and interests.

Although, to date, the principles of computed tomography have been applied primarily to the manipulation of x-ray transmission data, application of these principles to other imaging modalities has not escaped attention. Additional applications, encompassing the medical imaging disciplines of nuclear medicine (emission computed tomography), ultrasound, and nuclear magnetic resonance, are presented in the final chapters of the book. Development of these applications is one of the more promising arenas for future research efforts in diagnostic imaging.

W. R. H.

The Physical Principles of
Computed Tomography

1 Evolution of X-Ray Transmission Computed Tomography

HISTORICAL BACKGROUND

In the 1970s, x-ray transmission computed tomography (CT) entered the medical imaging arena with an impact that is perhaps unparalleled in the history of radiology. Because of the rapidity with which this imaging technique has been integrated into clinical medicine, and because of the significant improvements that have occurred in the very few years since CT was introduced, it is easy to believe that the principles of computed tomography are a relatively recent development. Actually, these principles evolved from the work of the Austrian mathematician J. Radon, who described the mathematics of reconstruction imaging in 1917 [16]. Radon's derivation of a solution to the mathematical problems of image reconstruction was unrelated to the production of images; he was working at the time on equations involving gravitational fields.

The development of reconstruction techniques as an imaging tool occurred primarily in two disciplines outside medicine. One of these was solar astronomy, in which image reconstruction techniques were used to produce a map of the emission of microwave radiation from the surface of the sun [5, 6]. Reconstruction imaging also was applied to electron micrography, in which electron transmission images were obtained as the specimen was rotated in the electron beam [9, 10]. From these transmission images, displays of the structure of complex molecules could be reconstructed. Techniques of image reconstruction also were applied to a variety of optical problems [4, 17].

The potential of reconstruction tomography as a clinical imaging technique was recognized first by W. H. Oldendorf. In 1961, Oldendorf [15] constructed a prototype CT scanner consisting of an iodine-131 radioactive source and a scintillation detector with the object rotating between the source and detector. A reproduction of Oldendorf's proposed design of a CT scanner is shown in Figure 1-1.

In the early 1960s, D. E. Kuhl and R. Q. Edwards devoted considerable effort to adapting the technique of image reconstruction from projections to problems in nuclear medicine. In 1963, these authors described the first attempt at emission CT [12, 13]. Later, Kuhl and co-workers developed a transmission tomography system employing an americium-241 source. In their early efforts, these investigators employed rather simplistic reconstruction mathematics, and the resulting images were not very clear. Nevertheless, Kuhl and Edwards are the undisputed orginators of the technique of emission computed tomography discussed later in this text.

In 1956 A. M. Cormack, a physicist at the University of Capetown, became interested in determining corrections for body inhomogeneities in patients scheduled for radiation therapy. These corrections required accurate values of attenuation coefficients across anatomic planes through the patient. Cormack realized that a cross-sectional matrix of coefficients could be determined if measurements of x-ray transmission were obtained at many angles and projections through the body. He realized also that these coefficients could be displayed as a gray-scale image of internal anatomy.

To explore the feasibility of the reconstruction approach to visualization of internal anatomy, Cormack assembled a 7 mCi cobalt-60 source and a Geiger-Müller (G-M) detector on opposite sides of a platform on which an aluminum and wood specimen was positioned. Data

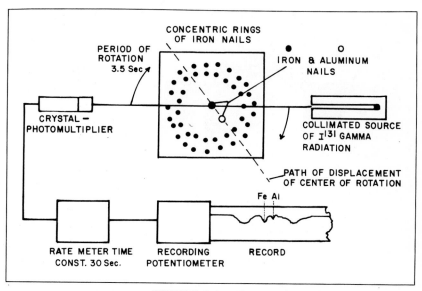

FIGURE 1-1.   *Prototype design of a CT scanner described by W. H. Oldendorf in 1961. (Reprinted from W. H. Oldendorf, Isolated flying spot detection of radiodensity discontinuities—displaying the internal structural pattern of a complex object.* IRE Trans. Bio-Med. Elect. *BME-8:68, 1961. With permission.)*

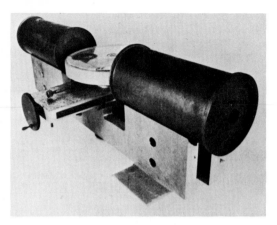

FIGURE 1-2. *Experimental apparatus used by Cormack in 1963 to obtain x-ray attenuation data for a nonsymmetric test object. (Reprinted from A. Cormack, Development of the CT Concept. In G. D. Fullerton and J. A. Zagzebski {eds.}*, Medical Physics of CT and Ultrasound: Tissue Imaging and Characterization. *New York: American Institute of Physics, 1980. P. 9. With permission.)*

on the transmission of ^{60}Co gamma rays at 5 mm increments were processed manually to yield the attenuation coefficients of the specimen as a function of radius. These results agreed well with the known composition of the phantom.

In 1957, Cormack moved to Tufts University in Boston, and his experimental work on reconstruction tomography was not revived until 1963. At that time, he repeated his experiment using a nonsymmetrical phantom and a computer for processing the transmission data obtained at 7½-degree angular increments. The experimental apparatus for these measurements, shown in Figure 1-2, was assembled at a cost of less than $100. The results of Cormack's 1956 and 1963 experiments were published in the physics literature, in which they received very little notice for a number of years [7, 8]. In 1979, Cormack (together with G. Hounsfield) was awarded the Nobel Prize in physiology and medicine for his pioneering work in reconstruction tomography.

In the late 1960s and early 1970s, a number of other investigators were exploring various approaches to reconstruction tomography as potential imaging techniques or as possible aids to treatment planning in radiation therapy. Among these investigators were O. J. Tretiak, M. Eden, and W. Simon [18] and R. H. T. Bates and T. M. Peters [3]. The principal breakthrough in reconstruction imaging, however, was the work of Hounsfield, an engineer at the Central Research Laboratories of Electro-Musical Instruments (EMI), Ltd., in England.

Hounsfield agreed with Cormack that images of the interior of the body could be reconstructed from a number of x-ray transmission measurements obtained tomographically. He concluded that attenuation coefficients could be computed to a theoretical accuracy of 0.5 percent and that these computations would not require exposing the patient to excessive levels of radiation. On the basis of these encouraging

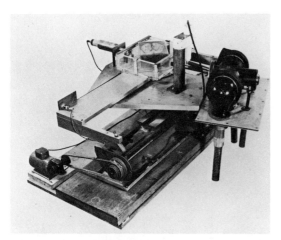

FIGURE 1-3.   *Early laboratory prototype of x-ray transmission CT scanner developed by Hounsfield. (Reprinted with permission of EMI, Ltd.)*

conclusions, Hounsfield assembled a model CT scanner consisting of a ^{241}Am source and sodium iodide detector. The source and detector were positioned on opposite sides of a motorized lathe bed that could undergo both translational and rotational motion. With this device Hounsfield was able to generate reconstruction data describing nonsymmetrical test objects. However, accumulation of the transmission data required nine days. To obtain a more intense source of radiation so that the time to collect data could be reduced, the radioactive source soon was replaced by an x-ray tube. The resulting apparatus is shown in Figure 1-3. With this apparatus and the help of two radiologists, J. Ambrose and L. Kreel, images were obtained of a variety of biologic specimens, including preserved human brain, fresh bullock brain, and pig carcass.

The first computed tomographic scanner for clinical scanning of the human head was installed in 1971 at the Atkinson Morley's Hospital in Wimbledon. The scanner employed synchronous translation of the x-ray source and NaI detector, with each translation occurring in a separate angular increment of 1 degree over a 180-degree arc. A water bag was positioned around the patient's skull to make the x-ray transmission path equal in all directions. A total of 28,800 transmission measurements was obtained over a period of 4½ minutes followed by another 20 minutes for image reconstruction. A photograph of an early clinical model of the EMI head scanner is shown in Figure 1-4.

In April 1972, clinical CT data obtained in Wimbledon were presented at the annual meeting of the British Institute of Radiology. The following day (April 21, 1972), a report on the scanner appeared in the *London Times*. Later in the same year, similar data were presented at the International Congress of Radiology and the Radiological Society of North America. Clinical data were first published in 1973 [2, 11]. In the summer of the same year, the first five commer-

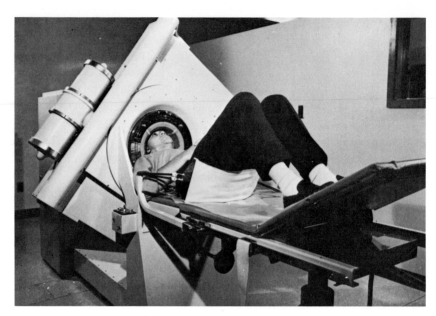

FIGURE 1-4. *Early clinical model of the first-generation EMI CT head scanner. (Reprinted with permission of EMI, Ltd.)*

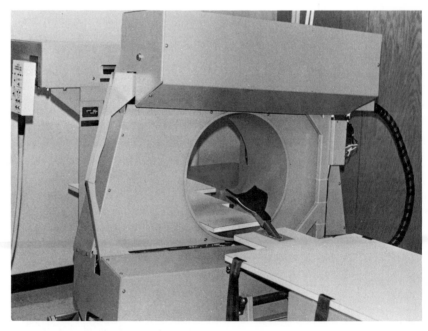

FIGURE 1-5. *Early clinical model of the first generation ACTA scanner. (Reprinted with permission of Pfizer, Inc.)*

cial EMI head scanners were installed in hospitals in London (National Hospital, Queen Square); Manchester, England; Glasgow; Rochester, Minnesota (Mayo Clinic); and Boston, Massachusetts (Massachusetts General Hospital).

As the EMI head scanner was being introduced into clinical medicine, R. S. Ledley of Georgetown University was developing the ACTA CT scanner for whole body as well as head examinations [14]. The first commercial model of the ACTA scanner was installed at the University of Minnesota in 1973. A photograph of this unit is reproduced in Figure 1-5.

At the Cleveland Clinic in 1974, the prototype of the Ohio Nuclear (now Technicare, Inc.) CT Delta Scanner was evaluated clinically by R. J. Alfidi and his associates [1]. This instrument employed a small fan-shaped array of multiple x-ray beams in place of the pencil x-ray beam used in the EMI and ACTA scanners. Because of this beam shape and the resulting reduction in patient examination time, the Delta scanner was the first unit to be categorized as a "second-generation" CT scanner. In 1974, the first third-generation CT scanner was introduced by General Electric Company. This scanner, which employed rotational motion only, was capable of collecting transmission data for a single image in as short a time as five seconds. One year later, the stationary detector array scanner was announced by American Science and Engineering and was labeled as the fourth generation in the evolution of computed tomographic scanners.

REFERENCES

1. Alfidi, R. J., et al. Experimental studies to determine application of CAT scanning to the human body. *Am. J. Roentgenol.* 124:199, 1975.
2. Ambrose, J. Computerized transverse axial scanning (tomography). II. Clinical application. *Br. J. Radiol.* 46:1023, 1973.

3. Bates, R. H. T., and Peters, T. M. Towards improvements in tomography. *N. Z. J. Sci.* 14:883, 1971.

4. Berry, M. V., and Gibbs, D. F. The interpretation of optical projections. *Proc. Roy. Soc.* A 314:143, 1970.

5. Bracewell, R. N. Strip integration in radio astronomy. *Aust. J. Phys.* 9:198, 1956.

6. Branson, N. J. B. A. The emission spectrum of the Crab Nebula. *Observatory* 85:250, 1965.

7. Cormack, A. M. Representation of a function by its line integrals, with some radiological applications. *J. Appl. Phys.* 34:2722, 1963.

8. Cormack, A. M. Representation of a function by its line integrals, with some radiological applications. II. *J. Appl. Phys.* 35:2908, 1964.

9. De Rosier, D. J., and Klug, A. Reconstruction of three-dimensional structures from electron micrographs. *Nature* 217:130, 1968.

10. Gordon, R., Bender, R., and Herman, G. T. Algebraic reconstruction techniques (ART) for three-dimensional electron microscopy and x-ray photography. *J. Theor. Biol.* 29:471, 1970.

11. Hounsfield, G. N. Computerized transverse axial scanning (tomography). I. Description of system. *Br. J. Radiol.* 46:1016, 1973.

12. Kuhl, D. E., and Edwards, R. Q. Image separation radioisotope scanning. *Radiology* 80:653, 1963.

13. Kuhl, D. E., Edwards, R. Q., Ricci, A. R., and Reivich, M. Quantitative section scanning using orthogonal tangent correction. *J. Nucl. Med.* 14:196, 1973.

14. Ledley, R. S., et al. Computerized transaxial x-ray tomography of the human body. *Science* 186:207, 1974.

15. Oldendorf, W. H. Isolated flying spot detection of radiodensity discontinuities—displaying the internal structural pattern of a complex object. *IRE Trans. Bio-Med. Elect.* BME-8:68, 1961.

16. Radon, J. *Über die Bestimmung von Funktionen durch ihre integralwerte längs gewisser Mannigfaltigkeiten. Saechsische Akademie der Wissenschaften, Leipzig. Berichte über die Verhandlungen* 69:262, 1917. [Translation by Analogic Corp., 1976: On the determination of functions by their integral values along certain manifolds.]

17. Rowley, P. D. Quantitative interpretation of three-dimensional weakly refractive phase objects using holographic interferometry. *J. Opt. Soc. Am.* 59:1496, 1969.

18. Tretiak, O. J., Eden, M., and Simon, W. *Internal Structure from X-Ray Images.* Proceedings of the Eighth International Conference on Medical and Biological Engineering, IEEE, Chicago, 1969.

X-Ray Attenuation Coefficients of Tissues

As a beam of x rays traverses a medium, it is attenuated by various absorption and scattering processes. Consequently, the intensity of the x-ray beam decreases with depth in the medium. For x-ray beams in the energy range used in computed tomography (CT), three interaction processes influence the rate of attenuation of the x-ray beam. These processes are coherent scattering, photoelectric absorption, and Compton interactions.

ABSORPTION AND SCATTERING PROCESSES

Coherent Scattering

In coherent scattering (also referred to as *Rayleigh* or *classical scattering*), an x ray is scattered from its original direction with negligible loss of energy. The scattering occurs as the x ray interacts with the electrons of an atom collectively, and the x ray usually is scattered through a rather narrow angle with respect to the direction of the incident x ray. Coherent scattering is a dominant interaction only for very low-energy x rays and occurs infrequently with the high–kilovolt peak (kVp), highly filtered x-ray beams used in CT. Coherent scattering is illustrated in Figure 2-1.

Photoelectric Absorption

In a photoelectric interaction, the entire energy of an x ray is transferred to an inner electron in an atom of the medium. The x ray disappears as its energy is transferred to the electron. The electron is ejected from the atom with a kinetic energy, E_K, which equals the x-ray energy, E_X, minus the binding energy, E_B, of the electron:

$$E_K = E_X - E_B.$$

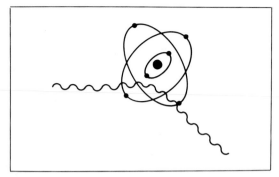

FIGURE 2-1. *Coherent scattering in which an x ray is scattered with negligible energy loss after interaction with the cloud of electrons in an atom.*

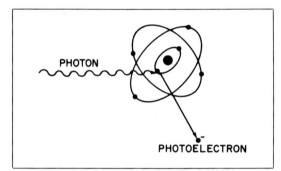

FIGURE 2-2. *Photoelectric interaction in which the energy of the x ray is transferred completely to an electron. The electron (termed a* photoelectron*) is ejected from the atom with a kinetic energy* $E_K = E_X - E_B$. *(Reproduced with permission from W. R. Hendee, Interactions of X and Gamma Rays.* Medical Radiation Physics: Roentgenology, Nuclear Medicine, and Ultrasound [2nd ed.]. *Chicago: Year Book, 1979. Chap. 6. Copyright © 1979 by Year Book Medical Publishers, Inc., Chicago.)*

The ejected electron is termed a *photoelectron*. For x rays in the energy range used in CT, the photoelectron is ejected at a relatively wide angle with respect to the incident x ray. The ejected electron creates a vacancy in the electron structure of the atom that gives rise to characteristic radiation and Auger electrons. A photoelectric interaction is illustrated in Figure 2-2.

The probability of photoelectric interaction decreases rapidly with increasing x-ray energy. This relationship, often described as a $1/E_X^3$ dependence of interaction probability on x-ray energy, is illustrated in Figure 2-3 for tissue constituents and for iodine. In the curve for iodine, discontinuities occur at energies corresponding to the binding energies of electrons in the K- and L-electron shells of iodine. At these energies, the x-ray energy is sufficient to eject electrons from the corresponding shell of the iodine atom, and the probability of interaction increases markedly.

For x rays that are absorbed photoelectrically, the probability of interaction increases rapidly with increasing atomic number of the absorbing medium. For this reason, the curve for iodine in Figure 2-3 is positioned above the curve for the tissue constituents—fat, muscle, and bone. The dependence of photoelectric interactions on atomic number is often described as a Z^3 dependence. In actuality, the dependence of interaction probability per unit mass of material varies about as $Z^{3.58}$ rather than Z^3.

In muscle, photoelectric absorption is the dominant interaction for x rays less than about 35 keV in energy. Above 35 keV, x rays tend to interact more frequently by Compton scattering than by photoelectric absorption.

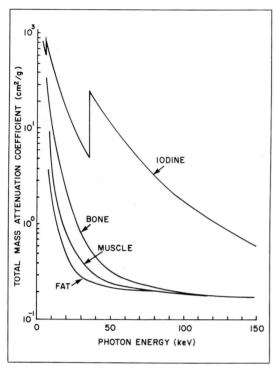

FIGURE 2-3. *Mass attenuation coefficient for iodine and various tissue constituents as a function of x-ray energy. For illustration purposes, the attenuation coefficient curve may be considered qualitatively as resembling the curve for probability of interaction.*

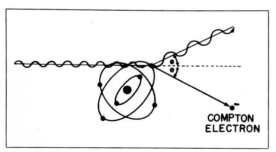

FIGURE 2-4. *Compton scattering of an x ray in which part of the incident x-ray energy is transferred to an electron of an absorbing atom. The remainder of the incident x-ray energy is retained by the scattered x ray. (Reproduced with permission from W. R. Hendee, Interactions of X and Gamma Rays.* Medical Radiation Physics: Roentgenology, Nuclear Medicine, and Ultrasound *[2nd ed.].* Chicago: Year Book, 1979. Chap. 6. Copyright © 1979 by Year Book Medical Publishers, Inc., Chicago.)

Compton Scattering

For x rays in the upper range of energies used in CT, the dominant interaction is Compton scattering. In this interaction, the x ray usually interacts with an outer electron of an atom of the medium. Part of the x ray's energy is imparted to the electron, and the electron is ejected from the atom with some amount of kinetic energy. The x ray is scattered in a new direction with reduced energy. If these scattered x rays are recorded during the image-forming process, they interfere with the visualization of detail in the image. For this reason, the scattered photons are rejected by a narrow collimator placed between the patient and the radiation detector. The characteristics of this collimating device are described in Chapter 4. A diagram of the Compton scattering process is shown in Figure 2-4.

Compton interactions occur predominantly with outer, essentially "unbound," electrons of an absorbing medium. The probability of Compton interactions increases with the number of these electrons per unit volume of absorber. That is, the probability of a Compton interaction increases with the electron density (electrons per gram) and with the physical density (g/cm^3) of the medium. The principal influence on electron density is the amount of hydrogen in a medium. This strong influence of hydrogen occurs because the electron density of hydrogen is two or more times the electron density of any other element. The electron density of hydrogen is greater because the common isotopic form of this element contains no neutrons. Therefore there is one electron for every nuclear particle in hydrogen, whereas in other elements there is one electron for every two or more nuclear particles.

For a high-kVp, heavily filtered x-ray beam such as that used in CT, almost all interactions in muscle and other soft tissues occur by Compton scattering. Only in higher Z materials such as bone and contrast agents containing barium and iodine are interactions by photoelectric processes significant.

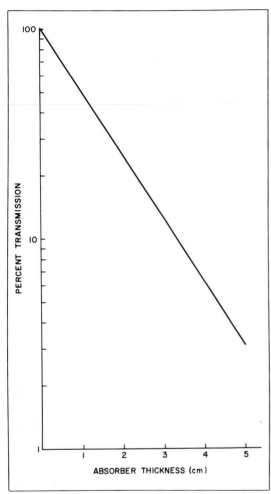

FIGURE 2-5. *Semilogarithmic plot of the transmission of a narrow beam of monoenergetic x rays as a function of thickness of an attenuating medium. (Reproduced with permission from W. R. Hendee, Interactions of X and Gamma Rays. Medical Radiation Physics: Roentgenology, Nuclear Medicine, and Ultrasound [2nd ed.]. Chicago: Year Book, 1979. Chap. 6. Copyright © 1979 by Year Book Medical Publishers, Inc., Chicago.)*

ATTENUATION OF AN X-RAY BEAM

The number of x rays attenuated in a medium depends on the number of x rays incident. This relationship is expressed as $P = \mu I$, where P is the rate of removal of x rays from the beam by absorption and scattering, I is the number of incident x rays, and μ is the attenuation coefficient of the medium for the x rays. If the rate of removal P is expressed per unit pathlength of x rays through the medium, then μ has units of 1/length and is known as the *linear attenuation coefficient*. If all the x rays in the beam have the same energy (i.e., the beam is monoenergetic), and if the beam is narrow and contains no scattered x rays, then the number I of x rays penetrating a medium of thickness x is $I = I_0 e^{-\mu x}$, where I_0 is the number of x rays incident on the medium. A semilogarithmic plot of I as a function of thickness x yields a straight line, as shown in Figure 2-5.

In transmission CT, monoenergetic radiation seldom is used, because it is available only from radioactive nuclides, and these sources lack the intensity required to produce useful images during short exposure times. Instead, x-ray beams from x-ray tubes are employed, and these beams contain a spectrum of x-ray energies up to a maximum value defined by the kVp applied to the tube. The transmission I of a polyenergetic x-ray beam through a thin slab of medium of thickness x is described as

$$I = I_0(E_1)e^{-\mu(E_1)x} + I_0(E_2)e^{-\mu(E_2)x} + \ldots + I_0(E_n)e^{-\mu(E_n)x}$$

In this expression $I_0(E_1)$, $I_0(E_2)$, etc. represent the incident intensities for each of n different x-ray energies present in the beam, and $\mu(E_1)$,

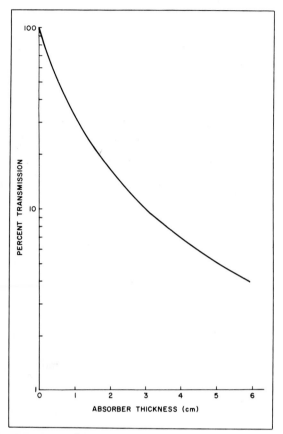

FIGURE 2-6. *Semilogarithmic plot of the transmission of a narrow beam of polyenergetic x rays as a function of absorber thickness.*

$\mu(E_2)$, etc. represent the linear attenuation coefficients appropriate for each of the n different energies. In shorthand notation, this expression may be written

$$I = \sum_{K=1}^{n} I_0(E_K)e^{-\mu(E_K)x}.$$

where K successively assumes each of several values from 1 to n, and Σ indicates that the expression computed with K set to a particular value is to be added to all the expressions computed with K less than the value. In general, the attenuation coefficient $\mu(E_K)$ is greater for x rays of lower energy, so that, as the beam penetrates the medium, the lower-energy x rays are selectively removed. Hence, the average energy of the x-ray beam increases with depth in the medium. This gradual increase in energy causes a semilogarithmic plot of x-ray transmission as a function of absorber thickness to depart from a straight line (Figure 2-6). This change in x-ray beam energy with depth results in the beam-hardening artifact characteristic of transmission CT images. This artifact is discussed in Chapter 10.

In many instances, including the mathematical reconstruction of images in CT, it is convenient to describe a polyenergetic x-ray beam in terms of its effective energy. The *effective energy* of an x-ray beam is the energy of a monoenergetic beam of photons (x rays or gamma rays) that would undergo the same attenuation in the medium as that experienced by the actual x-ray beam. To determine the effective energy, the fractional transmission I/I_0 of x rays through a thin medium of thickness x is measured, and from this measurement an effective linear attenuation coefficient μ is computed from the expression $I/I_0 = e^{-\mu x}$.

Next, the single x-ray energy that corresponds to this value of μ for the particular medium is determined from tabulated or measured data. This single x-ray energy is the effective energy of the polyenergetic x-ray beam. For CT scanners operating around 120 to 140 kVp, the effective energy usually is 70 to 80 keV.

The thickness of a medium that reduces the intensity of an x-ray beam to half is the *half-value layer* (HVL) of the medium for the x-ray beam. For x-ray beams used in CT, the HVL typically is 4 to 5 mm of aluminum.

ATTENUATION COEFFICIENTS AND CT NUMBERS

During the image-reconstruction process, the CT number computed for a material is related to the linear attenuation coefficient μ of the material for the effective energy of the x-ray beam. This relationship is indicated by the expression

$$\text{CT number} = \text{Constant} \left[\frac{\mu - \mu_w}{\mu_w} \right]$$

where μ_w is the linear-attenuation coefficient of water at the same effective energy [2]. For CT scanners of recent vintage, the constant in this expression has the value 1,000, and the CT numbers are referred to as *Hounsfield units* (HU). The expression for Hounsfield units is

$$\text{HU} = 1,000 \left[\frac{\mu - \mu_w}{\mu_w} \right] = 1,000 \frac{\mu}{\mu_w} - 1,000$$

In Hounsfield units, air has a value of $-1,000$; water has a value of 0; dense bone has a value of some hundreds of Hounsfield units; and metal, such as that used in surgical clips, may have HU values exceeding 1,000. In earlier scanners, the constant had other values (for example, in early EMI scanners, the constant had a value of 500).

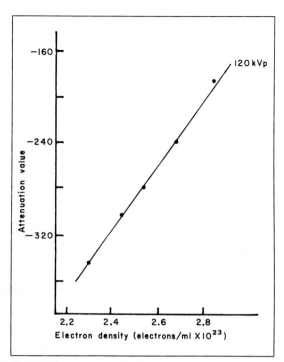

FIGURE 2-7.   *Linear relationship between CT number (Hounsfield units) and the volume electron density (electrons/cm³) of selected liquid hydrocarbons. (Modified from B. R. Pullan, R. G. Ritchings, and I. Isherwood, Accuracy and Meaning of Computed Tomography Attenuation Values. In T. H. Newton and D. G. Potts {eds.}, Radiology of the Skull and Brain: Technical Aspects of Computed Tomography, St. Louis: Mosby, 1981. Vol. 5, Chap. 111. With permission.)*

Because CT numbers are expressed as the ratio of attenuation coefficients between a material and water, they do not vary greatly with changes in kVp or filtration of the x-ray beam. Also, they remain relatively constant from one CT scanner to another. The major influences on CT numbers are the physical characteristics of the absorbing materials, primarily the physical (mass) density of the material in units of g/cm^3. A secondary influence on the values of CT numbers is the mass electron density (electrons per gram) of the medium, since most interactions occur by Compton scattering and this mode of interaction varies with the mass electron density but not with the atomic number of the medium. The product of mass electron density (electrons per gram) and the physical density (g/cm^3) is termed the *volume electron density* of the medium in units of electrons/cm^3. The volume electron density usually completely characterizes the CT number of an absorbing material. The linear relationship between CT number and volume electron density is shown in Figure 2-7. With the exception of bone, all biological specimens follow this linear relationship almost exactly. In bone, a small but significant fraction of the interactions are photoelectric; and the atomic number of the material influences the likelihood of interaction. Hence, the CT number for bone deviates a few percent from the linear relationship depicted in Figure 2-7.

For any material exposed to a diagnostic x-ray beam, the linear attenuation coefficient is the sum of the coefficients describing coherent scattering (K), photoelectric absorption (τ), and Compton scattering (σ). That is, $\mu = K + \tau + \sigma$. White and Fitzgerald [5] have shown that this expression can be rewritten as

$$\mu = \rho_e(k_1 Z^{1.69} + k_2 Z^{3.58} + k_3 Z^{-0.03})$$

where ρ_e is the volume electron density in electrons/cm^3, and k_1, k_2, and k_3 are the fraction of interactions that occur by coherent scattering, photoelectric absorption, and Compton scattering, respectively. In most biological materials with the exception of dense bone, k_1 and k_2 are negligibly small and the effective atomic numbers are similar. Hence, the linear attenuation coefficient μ and, therefore, the corresponding CT number vary only with the volume electron density, as noted above.

The exact expression for μ described by White can be substituted in the expression HU = 1,000 μ/μ_w − 1,000 to yield "ideal" CT numbers. Listed in Table 2-1 are ideal CT numbers computed by Fullerton [1] for selected materials. These values suggest that a unique CT number exists for each biological constituent and that the numbers obtained for a specific tissue might be useful in characterizing the composition of the tissue and its normal or pathologic state. Tissue characterization by analysis of CT numbers is discussed in Chapter 11.

As was noted earlier, the volume electron density is primarily a reflection of the mass density in g/cm^3; that is, the mass electron density in units of electrons per gram exerts only a secondary influence on volume electron density. For most soft tissues, therefore, CT numbers should vary closely with the mass density of the absorbing material. This close correlation between CT number and mass density is shown in Figure 2-8 for a variety of soft tissues.

Table 2-1.   *Volume Electron Densities Compared to Water and Ideal CT Numbers for Human Soft Tissues at Selected Effective Energies for the CT X-Ray Beam*

Tissue/Organ	Relative Volume Electron Density	Ideal CT Number		
		62 keV (eff)	72 KeV (eff)	79 keV (eff)
Adipose	0.925	−114	−101	−94
Blood	1.054	58	56	56
Brain	1.033	38	36	36
Heart	1.024	24	24	24
Kidney	1.045	45	45	45
Muscle	1.054	59	57	56
Pancreas	1.048	48	48	48
Water	1.000	0	0	0

Source: Fullerton, G. D. Fundamentals of CT Tissue Characterization. In G. D. Fullerton and J. A. Zagzebski (eds.), *Medical Physics of CT and Ultrasound: Tissue Imaging and Characterization.* New York: American Institute of Physics, 1980. Pp. 125–162.

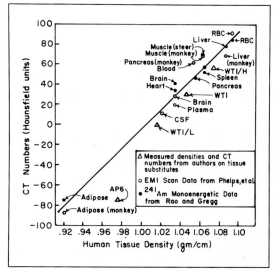

FIGURE 2-8.   *CT numbers measured for excised tissue samples by Phelps, Hoffman, and Ter-Pogossian {3} and Rao and Gregg {4}, and for tissue-simulating plastics by Fullerton {1}, plotted against best estimates of tissue and tissue-substitute mass densities. (Reprinted from G. D. Fullerton, Fundamentals of CT Tissue Characterization. In G. D. Fullerton and J. A. Zagzebski {eds.}, Med-*ical Physics of CT and Ultrasound: Tissue Imaging and Characterization. *New York: American Institute of Physics, 1980. P. 125. With permission.)*

In summary, the CT number of a tissue constituent varies directly with the linear attenuation coefficient μ of the constituent according to the relationship

$$CT\ number\ =\ Constant\ \frac{\mu\ -\ \mu_w}{\mu_w}$$

where μ_w is the linear attenuation coefficient of water. For CT numbers expressed in Hounsfield units, the constant has a value of 1,000. Since the linear attenuation coefficient varies directly with the volume electron density (electrons/cm^3) of biologic tissues (with the exception of bone), CT numbers for these tissues are a direct reflection of the volume electron density. The volume electron density is affected primarily by the physical density (g/cm^3) of tissue; hence, CT numbers are an index primarily of the physical densities of various tissue constituents and only secondarily reveal differences in mass electron density (electrons per gram) or atomic number.

REFERENCES

1. Fullerton, G. D. Fundamentals of CT Tissue Characterization. In G. D. Fullerton and J. A. Zagzebski (eds.), *Medical Physics of CT and Ultrasound: Tissue Imaging and Characterization.* New York: American Institute of Physics, 1980. Pp. 125–162.
2. McCullough, E. C. Photon attenuation in computed tomography. *Med. Phys.* 2:307, 1975.
3. Phelps, M. E., Hoffman, E. J., and Ter-Pogossian, M. M. Attenuation coefficients of various body tissues, fluid, and lesions at photon energies of 18 and 136 keV. *Radiology* 117:573, 1975.
4. Rao, P. S., and Gregg, E. C. Attenuation of monoenergetic gamma rays in tissues. *Am. J. Roentgenol.* 123:631, 1975.
5. White, D. R., and Fitzgerald, M. Calculated attenuation and energy-absorption coefficients for ICRP Reference Man (1975) organs and tissues. *Health Phys.* 33:73, 1977.

3 Four Generations of Computed Tomographic Scanners

In less than four years after the introduction of the first EMI CT unit in 1972, CT evolved through four generations of scanners. This rapid evolution was due primarily to improvements in the mechanical design of the scanners, which yielded shorter scan times and therefore better control over patient motion. Illustrated in Figure 3-1 is the reduction in scan time of CT scanners over the period from 1972 to 1977.

FIRST-GENERATION CT SCANNERS

The original first-generation CT scanner was the EMI unit installed in 1971 at Atkinson Morley's Hospital in Wimbledon. Later versions of this scanner were marketed by EMI as the Mark I scanner. The basic features of this scanner are diagrammed in Figure 3-2. This figure was included in the first article published by G. N. Hounsfield on the topic of computed tomography [1].

In the scanner depicted in Figure 3-2, the x-ray beam is collimated into two parallel pencil-like x-ray beams. These beams are directed toward two NaI scintillation detectors adjacent to each other on the opposite side of the patient. In this manner, transmission data can be collected simultaneously for two adjacent tomographic images of the patient's head. The x-ray tube, collimator, and detectors are part of a common frame that scans across the patient so that the x-ray tube and detectors move in synchrony on opposite sides of the patient. During this linear scanning motion, 240 measurements of x-ray transmission are obtained and compared to the x-ray transmission of water. This process is depicted by scan 1 in the scanning sequence diagram of Figure 3-3. When the scanner has reached the end of its translational motion, the frame is rotated through 1 degree and the process is repeated (scan 2 in Figure 3-3). The sec-

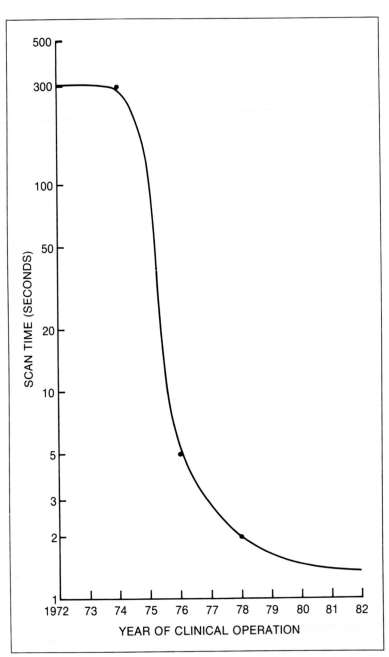

FIGURE 3-1. *Single-image collection time for the ten-year period after the introduction of CT scanners.*

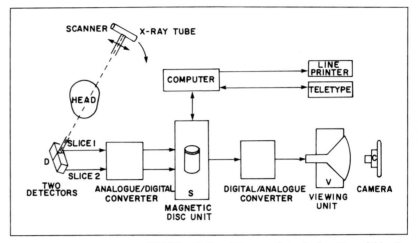

FIGURE 3-2.   *Diagram from the first Hounsfield publication on computed tomography. This diagram describes how signals from two detectors are digitized, stored on a magnetic disk, processed by computer and printed on a line printer. The signals also can be displayed as an image on the viewing unit. (Reprinted from G. N. Hounsfield, Computerized transverse axial scanning (tomography). I. Description of system.* Br. J. Radiol. *46:1016, 1973. With permission.)*

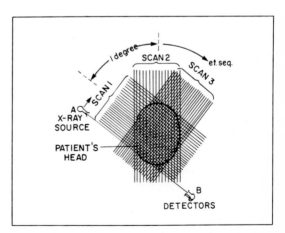

FIGURE 3-3.   *Scanning sequence of a first generation computed tomographic scanner. (Reprinted from G. N. Hounsfield, Computerized transverse axial scanning (tomography). I. Description of system.* Br. J. Radiol. *46:1016, 1973. With permission.)*

ond scan adds 240 measurements of x-ray transmission to those accumulated during the first scan. At the end of each translational scan, the rotation through 1 degree is repeated until the frame has rotated through 180 degrees. The scanning process yields a total of 240 transmission measurements per degree times 180 degrees, or 43,200 transmission measurements for each tomographic image.

To correct for varying x-ray intensity during the scanning process, a separate detector is positioned to the side of the pencil-like x-ray beam (Figure 3-4). This detector monitors the intensity of the x-ray beam, and its signal is used to correct transmission readings for fluctuating x-ray intensity.

The x-ray transmission measurements are delivered to a computer, which generates a set of simultaneous equations equal in number to the number of transmission measurements. From these equations, a series of CT numbers is computed to be displayed as a gray scale image on the display unit. In the first CT scanner, the display unit provided an 80 × 80 matrix of 6,400 viewing elements (called *picture elements,* or *pixels*). As long as there are more equations than pixels, a distinct CT number can be computed for each pixel. Since there are 43,200 equations, this requirement is satisfied so long as the number of pixels remains at 6,400. In fact, a matrix as fine as 160 × 160 (25,600 pixels) could be used without surpassing the number of equations and CT numbers available. Early in its marketing program, EMI substituted a 160 × 160 matrix for the 80 × 80 display unit.

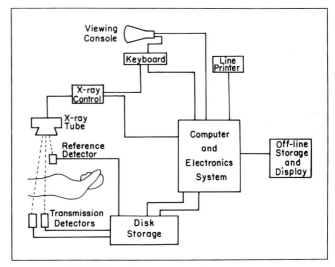

FIGURE 3-4.   *Diagram of a first-generation CT scanner illustrating the off-axis detector used to correct transmission readings for variable intensity of the x-ray beam.*

In early EMI first-generation scanners, the patient's head was positioned in a rubber cap with a circular orifice. With this technique, the entire path for x-ray transmission was filled by either water or the patient's head, and there was no air in the path of the x rays. Hence, the patient produced only small disturbances in the transmission of x rays through water, and the detector signals varied over a rather limited range. This limited range of detector response simplified the computations and improved the accuracy of CT numbers computed by early EMI scanners. In later scanners the water bags around the patient's head were discarded, and today no commerical scanners employ this technique.

In the original EMI first-generation scanner, data collection required $4\frac{1}{2}$ minutes and 5 minutes were needed to compute the CT numbers for a single image. The computations were performed while the scanner was accumulating data for the next tomographic image, and a total time of at least 35 minutes was required to accumulate and process the data for a six-image study of a patient. The exposure to the patient was on the order of 2 R or less, with the maximum exposure on the surface nearest the x-ray tube.

First-generation scanners, expecially those of more recent design, furnish images of reasonable quality that are satisfactory for many studies of the head. However, it is often difficult for patients to remain completely still during the long scanning process, and motion artifacts frequently are present in images made with first-generation scanners. In other regions of the body (e.g., the abdomen), where motion is more difficult to control, first-generation scanners are less than satisfactory. The first effort to improve scanner design was to reduce the time required to collect transmission data. This effort led to the second-generation CT scanner.

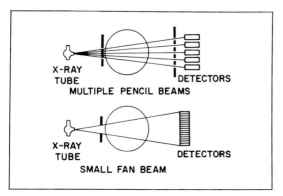

FIGURE 3-5.   *Multiple pencil-like x-ray beams in a fan-shaped geometry* (top) *and a fan-shaped x-ray beam* (bottom). *Both of these geometries are used in second-generation CT scanners. (Reprinted from R. A. Brooks, Comparative Evaluation of CT Scanner Technology. In G. D. Fullerton and J. A. Zagzebski {eds.}, Medical Physics of CT and Ultrasound: Tissue Imaging and Characterization. New York: American Institute of Physics, 1980. With permission.)*

SECOND-GENERATION CT SCANNERS

The adjacent detectors in the EMI first-generation scanner permit simultaneous collection of data for two adjacent tomographic sections, but they do not speed the data-accumulation process for a single section. Other manufacturers recognized that increased speed could be gained by placing the detectors side by side in the same scan plane rather than in adjacent scan planes. In the first application of this geometry, three detectors are placed side by side and receive three pencil-like x-ray beams in a fan-shaped pattern. With this approach, the x-ray tube and detector frame can be rotated 3 degrees, rather than 1 degree, at the end of each translational motion, and the data accumulation time is reduced by a factor of about 2. Subsequent developments have led to as many as 52 detectors in the scan plane and, in some second-generation scanners, two sets of multiple detectors to yield simultaneous measurements of transmission data in two adjacent scan planes. As more detectors were added, it became increasingly difficult to maintain the alignment of each pencil x-ray beam in the fan-shaped geometry. To overcome this difficulty, a continuous fan of x rays was substituted for the pencil-like x-ray beams, and each detector was collimated to accept only x rays along a line extending from the x-ray target. The fan-beam geometry irradiated a greater volume of tissue, and more scattered radiation was produced. The detectors had to be shielded from this scattered radiation. Also, the detectors had to be balanced carefully so that they were all equally sensitive to the impinging radiation. The pencil-beam fan-shaped geometry and the fan x-ray beam are illustrated in Figure 3-5.

With a fan-shaped x-ray beam and multiple detectors moving in the translate-rotate geometry characteristic of second-generation CT scanners, data collection times for a single tomographic section were reduced initially to as

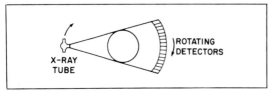

RROTATING
DETECTORS

X-RAY
TUBE

FIGURE 3-6.   *A third-generation computed tomo-graphic scanner employing purely rotational motion. (Reprinted from R. A. Brooks, Comparative Evaluation of CT Scanner Technology. In G. D. Fullerton and J. A. Zagzebski {eds.},* Medical Physics of CT and Ultrasound: Tissue Imaging and Characterization. *New York: American Institute of Physics, 1980. With permission.)*

little as 20 seconds and later to 5.3 seconds. However, even scan times as short as 20 seconds are too long for studies of abdominal structures, in which motion is extremely difficult to control, especially in ill patients who are unable to suspend respiration for this period of time. Further efforts to reduce scan time led to the third generation of CT scanners.

THIRD-GENERATION CT SCANNERS

With second-generation CT scanners, scan times still are limited by the need to move the x-ray tube and detectors through two degrees of motion, translational and rotational. By simplifying the motion solely to rotation such that the x-ray tube and detectors simply rotate around the patient, with no translational motion whatsoever, scan times can be reduced even further. This simplification in scanning geometry was announced in 1975 by General Electric (GE) Company as a third-generation computed tomographic scanner. With the GE scanner, data collection times for a single image are reduced to as little as 4.8 seconds, and even shorter times (down to 2.5 seconds) are available with other commercial versions of third-generation scanners. Modern versions of the third-generation CT scanner employ over 500 detectors extending over an arc between 21 and 45 degrees on the side of the patient opposite the x-ray tube. By shifting the array of detectors so that they are slightly misaligned with respect to the center of rotation of the detectors and x-ray tube, the number of independent measurements of x-ray transmission can be increased by a factor of 2 or more, and the quality of images obtained with third-generation scanners can be improved. A diagram of a third-generation scanner is shown in Figure 3-6.

In a third-generation scanner, most of the detectors are always in the shadow of the patient during an examination, and the response of the

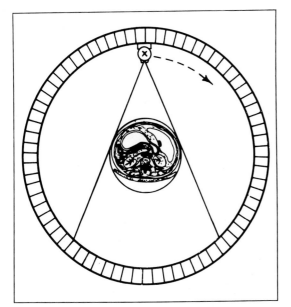

FIGURE 3-7.   *A fourth-generation computed tomographic scanner with a stationary ring of scintillation detectors and an x-ray tube that rotates around the patient. (Reprinted from W. R. Hendee, History of Computed Tomography. In G. D. Fullerton and J. A. Zagzebski {eds.},* Medical Physics of CT and Ultrasound: Tissue Imaging and Characterization. *New York: American Institute of Physics, 1980. With permission.)*

detectors cannot be normalized during a scan. Consequently, images from a third-generation scanner conceivably could be subject to artifacts caused by detector imbalance. Through the use of stable detectors and electronics, however, detector imbalance in third-generation scanners has not been a significant problem.

FOURTH-GENERATION SCANNERS

By 1974, many commercial organizations and institutional laboratories were attempting to design and build a CT scanner. The National Institutes of Health (NIH) of the United States Department of Health, Education, and Welfare (now the Department of Health and Human Services) became concerned that these efforts were not being monitored by any peer review process to ensure realization of the optimum design for a CT scanner. To eliminate this potential problem, NIH announced the availability of a competitive contract for the optimum design of a CT scanner. The contract was awarded to American Science and Engineering Company (AS & E), a small company in Cambridge, Massachusetts, that had previously been best known for its baggage x-ray systems for airports. Two years later, AS & E announced the fourth-generation design of a CT scanner.

In the AS & E design, more than 600 scintillation detectors are positioned side by side to form a ring that completely surrounds the patient. These detectors remain stationary while the x-ray tube rotates inside the ring and around the patient's body (Figure 3-7). With this scanning geometry, data for a single image can be collected in as short a time as 2 seconds. Another advantage of the fourth-generation design is receipt of the unattenuated x-ray beam by each detector twice during each scan. This unattenuated beam can be used to normalize the response of each detector, to prevent image artifacts caused by detector imbalance. The major disadvantages of the fourth-generation design are

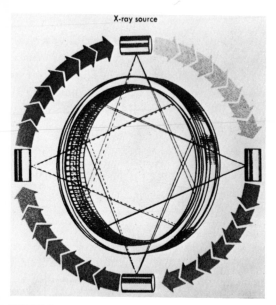

X-ray source

FIGURE 3-8. *Nutating geometry employed in the fourth-generation scanner designed by EMI, Ltd. (EMI Model 7070). A nonrotating ring of detectors is positioned near the patient and wobbles to permit entry of the x-ray beam from a tube rotating around and outside the detector ring. (Reprinted from L. M. Zatz, General Overview of Computed Tomography Instrumentation. In T. H. Newton and D. G. Potts {eds.},* Radiology of the Skull and Brain: Technical Aspects of Computed Tomography, *Vol. 5. St. Louis: Mosby, 1981. With permission.)*

the high cost associated with the large number of detectors (more than 2000 in some fourth-generation scanners), an increased susceptibility to scattered radiation, and unused primary radiation directed toward spaces separating the detectors. Because of this unused primary radiation, the radiation dose to the patient is usually greater for fourth-generation scanners than for third-generation scanners. These advantages and disadvantages counterbalance each other, so no particular clinical advantages are gained by the choice of a fourth-generation over a third-generation scanner, or vice versa.

A variation in design of fourth-generation CT scanners was conceived by EMI for its Model 7000 series of scanners. This design employs the concept of "nutating geometry," in which the x-ray tube is positioned slightly outside the ring of detectors (Figure 3-8). As the x-ray tube rotates around the ring of 1,088 detectors, the ring wobbles so that the fan-shaped x-ray beam can reach the patient without passing through the detectors. The principal advantage of this design is that x rays are utilized more efficiently because the detectors are closer to the patient.

A second variation in the design of fourth-generation scanners was proposed by Artronix, Inc. In this design, the x-ray tube is positioned at the center of a ring of 720 stationary detectors and rotates continuously about its axis through 360 degrees. Simultaneously with this rotation, the x-ray tube and circular array of detectors move in synchrony around the patient, without rotation of the detector ring. This approach is intended to optimize the use of primary radiation. Unfortunately, Artronix disappeared from the list of manufacturers of computed tomography units before the design could be evaluated clinically. The Artronix concept for optimum design of a CT scanner is illustrated in Figure 3-9.

A summary of the principal features of the four generations of CT scanners is provided in Table 3-1.

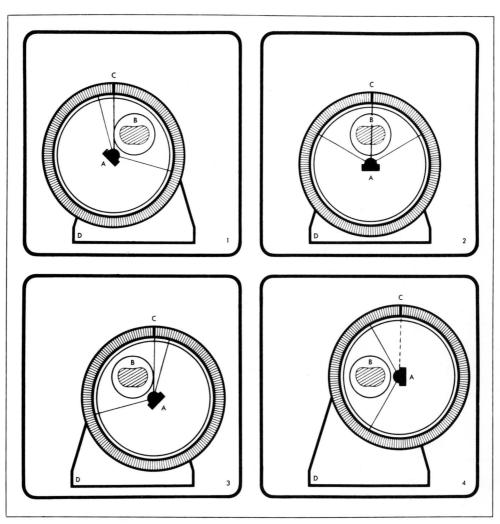

FIGURE 3-9.   *Configuration of the Artronix 1120 scanner in which the detector ring and x-ray tube move in synchrony around the patient as the x-ray tube rotates about its own axis. Steps in image formation are illustrated by the sequence of frames 1 to 4. (Reprinted from L. M. Zatz, General Overview of Computed Tomography Instrumentation. In T. H. Newton and D. G. Potts {eds.},* Radiology of the Skull and Brain: Technical Aspects of Computed Tomography, *Vol. 5. St. Louis: Mosby, 1981. With permission.)*

Table 3-1. *Characteristic Features of Four Generations of CT Scanners*

Feature	Generation			
	First	Second	Third	Fourth
X-ray tube and detector motion	Translate/rotate	Translate/rotate	Rotate only	Tube rotates/detectors stationary
Detectors per section	1	3–52	128–511	242–72,000
X-ray beam per section	Single pencil	Multiple pencil or narrow fan (3–26°)	Wide fan (21–45°)	Wide fan (48–120°)
Minimum scan time	4–5 min	5.3 sec–3.5 min	3–4.8 sec	1–5 sec

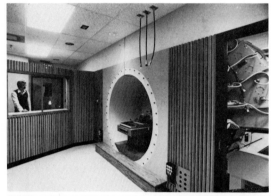

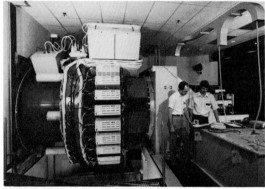

FIGURE 3-10. *The "Dynamic Spatial Reconstructor" under development at the Mayo Clinic (Rochester, Minnesota) employs 28 x-ray tubes and 28 light-amplifier TV chains to produce computed tomographic images in times as short as 100 msec. (Reproduced with permission from R. A. Robb, The dynamic spatial reconstructor: From basic concepts to applications. Fourth Symposium on Physical and Technical Aspects of Computed Tomography, Tokyo, September 1981.)*

FIFTH-GENERATION CT SCANNERS

The evolution of CT through four generations over a period of slightly more than four years is a reflection of improvements in mechanical design. These improvements led to simplifications in the scanning motion, until a purely rotational geometry had been achieved. Further reductions in scan time are limited more by the output of the x-ray tube than by the mechanical design of the scanner. To reduce scan times to the millisecond region, either a new design for x-ray tubes has to be conceived or multiple x-ray tubes that fire successively have to be employed. Both approaches are under development and are discussed in Chapter 13. A brief review of one scanner employing multiple x-ray tubes is presented here.

In the Dynamic Spatial Reconstructor under development at the Mayo Clinic in Rochester, Minnesota, 28 x-ray tubes are positioned around a semicircular gantry. The tubes are in line with 28 light amplifiers and TV cameras, which are placed behind a curved fluorescent screen that occupies the remaining semicircle. The geometry is diagrammed in Figure 3-10. The gantry of x-ray tubes and imaging systems is proposed to rotate continuously around the patient at 15 revolutions per minute. This rotation will yield a set of 28 data-collection views every 1/10 second, and up to 240 equally spaced data-collection views over 360 degrees in less than 2 seconds. In this manner, images will be produced for data collection times as short as 16 milliseconds.

INDUSTRIAL CASUALTIES ALONG THE WAY

In the race to improve the design of CT scanners and to capture a share of the commercial marketplace, industrial competition in CT has been exceptionally severe. Some companies that entered the commercial arena lacked the resources to stay abreast of the competition in development and market visibility. Other companies realized that their scanner design was inferior to others on the market. Some of these companies withdrew from the commercial CT arena and applied their resources to less competitive areas, while others totally expended their financial resources and collapsed. From 1976 to 1977, there were 20 or so companies in the CT marketplace; three years later there were only nine companies.

REFERENCE

1. Hounsfield, G. N. Computerized transverse axial scanning (tomography). I. Description of system. *Br. J. Radiol.* 46:1016, 1973.

4

Physical Characteristics of Computed Tomographic Scanners

Early computed tomographic (CT) scanners employed x-ray source and detector systems and data-processing electronics and viewing units that were traditionally used for other applications in physics research and medical imaging. As the market for CT units developed and the scanners became more sophisticated, many of the scanner components were selected or developed for specific application to computed tomography. Today, some of these developments are being used in other areas of medical imaging, thereby further enhancing the impact of computed tomography on the entire field of radiology.

X-RAY TUBES

First- and second-generation CT units employ an industrial-type x-ray tube with a stationary anode and a maximum load capacity of up to 5 kilowatts for continuous operation. This capacity is greater than that available with rotating anode x-ray tubes and is required for the long exposure times accompanying the translate/ rotate geometry. The targets are composed of tungsten embedded in a copper anode and provide a target angle of about 20 degrees. The projected focal spot is 1 to 4 mm in width and 10 to 20 mm in length, with the long axis of the focal spot perpendicular to the axis of the x-ray tube. The inherent filtration of the x-ray tube and the aluminum or copper filtration added to the beam to increase its penetration yield a total filtration equivalent to that provided by a 3 to 8 mm thickness of aluminum. The x-ray tubes are operated at nearly constant potential, to prevent changes in beam intensity and quality from one transmission measurement to the next.

In third- and fourth-generation CT scanners, x-ray tubes with stationary anodes have been replaced by tubes with rotating anodes. This replacement provides increased x-ray intensity during relatively short exposure times, and a reduction in focal spot size. To eliminate torque on the bearings of the anode shaft, the x-ray tube is mounted so that the anode spins in a plane perpendicular to the motion of the tube. Continuous scanning of a CT unit may be limited by the heat-storage capacity of the anode, and intervals may be required between successive series of scans to permit anode cooling.

In many of the faster scanners, the operation of the x-ray tube is pulsed to control the length of each time interval over which data are collected. This control is essential in most fast scanners because the x-ray tube moves continuously and the movement of the tube during each sampling interval must not exceed about 1 millimeter if spatial resolution is to be maintained. There are a number of other advantages with pulsed rotating anode x-ray tubes. These advantages are (1) more efficient use of x rays for a given tube loading, (2) elimination of unnecessary radiation exposure, (3) an increased number of x rays available for each transmission measurement, (4) simplification of the electronics associated with each detector, and (5) closer monitoring of detector signals. In a pulsed x-ray tube, the typical duty cycle (percentage of time the x-ray tube is on) is about 20 percent, and each pulse lasts 2 to 3 milliseconds at 600 mA maximum.

X-RAY DETECTORS

In earlier CT scanners, sodium iodide (NaI) detectors, operated in current mode, are used to record the transmission of x rays through the patient. These detectors are used widely in physics research and provide high efficiency for detection of x rays. However, NaI detectors have a few disadvantages that have made their application less desirable in the faster CT scanners which operate without a water bag. Among the disadvantages are (1) a nonlinear response for radiation of different intensities, (2) a limited dynamic range, and (3) an afterglow of the NaI crystal that could permit the emitted light to carry over from one sampling interval to the next. Two approaches have been taken to overcome the limitations of NaI detectors. The first is the identification of other scintillation detectors with improved properties compared to NaI. The second approach is the use of ionization chambers or solid-state devices in place of scintillation detectors.

Scintillation Detectors Other Than NaI

Two scintillation detectors have been identified as possessing properties superior to NaI for fast scanning techniques in CT. The first to be tried was calcium fluoride (CaF_2) doped with europium. This crystal is less efficient than NaI (e.g., at 70 keV, the detection efficiency is 62 percent for a 1-in.-thick CaF_2 crystal, and 80 percent for a 2-in.-thick CaF_2 crystal, compared to about 100 percent for a 1-in.-thick NaI crystal) [2, 7]. However, the afterglow of CaF_2 is negligible. A second scintillator that has been adopted widely is bismuth germanate (BGO). This scintillator exhibits very little afterglow, and its high density and effective atomic number provide an efficiency of almost 100 percent for stopping x rays of diagnostic quality. Its light output (amount of light released for a given amount of x-ray energy absorbed), however, is only about 12 percent of the light output from NaI. Nevertheless, BGO detectors are today the most popular scintillation detectors for CT scanners [3].

Some recent scanners employ scintillation detectors of cesium iodide (CsI doped with thallium) coupled to silicon photodiodes rather than to photomultiplier tubes, because the light sensitivity of the photodiodes is matched closely to the wavelengths of light emitted from CsI. One advantage of these solid-state detectors is that they can be fabricated in any size and shape. Furthermore, they can be packed close together. Expanded use of photodiode solid state detectors can be anticipated in CT scanners of the future.

Ionization Detectors

As an alternative to scintillation detectors, xenon-filled ionization chambers are used in some (primarily third-generation) CT scanners. To improve the x-ray detection efficiency of these devices, they are operated under high pressure (8–10 atm) in a long, narrow configuration, with the long axis pointed toward the x-ray tube. These detectors are about 60 percent efficient in absorbing diagnostic x rays [1, 8]. Gas-filled detectors are not used with fourth-generation scanners because the orientation of the fan-shaped x-ray beam changes with respect to the detectors as the x-ray tube sweeps around the patient. Xenon-filled ionization chambers have proved equal to scintillation detectors in their suitability for CT scanning. The lower cost of ionization chambers is a major advantage over scintillation detectors.

COLLIMATION

In a CT scanner, the detectors are operated in current mode, and pulse-height analysis cannot be used to reject scattered radiation from the patient. To reject scattered photons and to localize the field of view of the detector, a collimator must be positioned in front of each detector. In a sense, the detector collimators function like a radiographic grid in front of an intensifying screen. For a pencil-beam CT scanner, Judy [6] has estimated that less than 0.2 percent of the radiation reaching the detector is scattered radiation. This amount increases somewhat with fan-beam geometry.

In a third-generation scanner, the collimators are all pointed toward the x-ray tube, permitting maximum use of primary x rays. With a fourth-generation scanner, the collimators must be oriented toward the center of the patient because the x-ray tube moves with respect to the detectors. Hence, some of the primary photons are intercepted by the collimators as the x-ray tube sweeps around the patient. For this reason, fourth-generation CT scanners utilize x rays somewhat less efficiently than do other scanners.

The width of the collimator aperture and the distance scanned by the x-ray tube during a data-sampling interval are the primary influences on the spatial resolution of a computed tomographic image. For this reason, a display matrix composed of very small picture elements does not necessarily imply that the spatial resolution of the image is equally good, because the picture elements may be much smaller than the collimator aperture or scanning increment. It is conceivable that the x-ray beam might be sampled more than once as the beam sweeps across a distance equal to the aperture width. In this case, some improvement in spatial resolution might be obtained by subtracting successive transmission measurements. Image noise caused by limitations in the number of photons would be intensified, however, and commercial CT scanners have not employed this technique to date.

The aperture of the "prepatient" collimator between the x-ray tube and the patient determines the width of the tomographic slice viewed in the CT image. Most scanners have source collimators that can be varied manually or automatically to provide different slice thicknesses (from 1–15 mm). Thinner slices yield improved depth resolution (i.e., reduced "partial volume artifact") but only at the expense of increased noise in the image or of a higher dose to the patient. These relationships are discussed in Chapter 9.

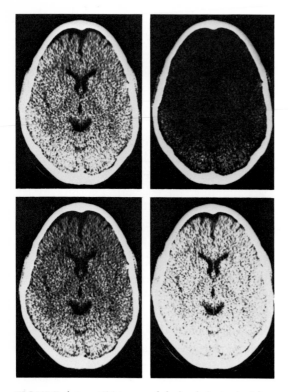

FIGURE 4-1. *CT images of the head obtained with constant window width but different settings of window level.*

VIEWING CONSOLE

After all the transmission measurements have been accumulated for a single tomographic image, a two-dimensional matrix of data is computed. These data are CT numbers that are related to x-ray attenuation coefficients in a cross-sectional plane through the patient. For most studies, the CT numbers are displayed as a gray-scale image on the viewing console. This console is either a television monitor or, less frequently, a storage oscilloscope with a long-persistence phosphor. In either case, the dynamic range of the display device (i.e., the number of shades of gray, or *gray scale*) is inadequate to encompass the entire range of CT numbers and still distinguish regions with slightly different CT numbers as different shades of gray. Usually, only a limited range of CT numbers is of interest in the image. To display this range of CT numbers, a window on the viewing console is employed to superimpose the limited gray scale over the range of CT numbers of interest. The number of shades of gray provided by the viewing console should be at least 32 and preferably 64 [9]. Although some CT units offer the option of a color display, this feature has not found wide clinical acceptance.

The range of CT numbers displayed in the image on the viewing console is determined by the "window width" control of the viewing window, and the CT number in the center of this range is determined by the "window level" control. Usually only one window is employed, although, for certain studies (e.g., those employing a contrast agent), two windows are sometimes used to superimpose contrast-containing structures on an image of normal anatomy. Images obtained at different settings of the viewing window are shown in Figures 4-1 and 4-2.

As an optional feature, most CT units offer a second, free-standing viewing console contain-

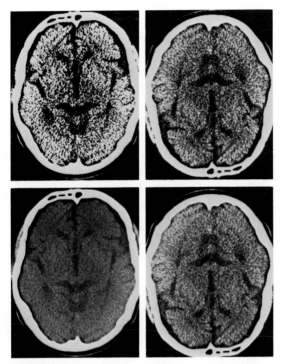

FIGURE 4-2. *CT images of the head obtained with constant window level but different settings of window width.*

ing its own computer and data-input devices. With this console, the physician can analyze data for previous patients without interrupting the examination of patients in the CT-unit gantry. Although relatively expensive, a free-standing physician's viewing console may be a worthwhile investment for busy CT facilities.

Most viewing consoles provide an image zoom feature, in which a limited region of anatomy can be viewed with variable magnification. The simplest approach to image zooming is electronic magnification in which the image is enlarged with no change in spatial resolution. This method is equivalent to viewing the image with a magnifying lens, and, although the image is enlarged, no improvement in spatial resolution is provided. With electronic magnification, data usually are interpolated to fill in some of the picture elements of the display so that the image is more pleasing to the eye.

Recently, some companies have introduced a zoom feature to improve spatial resolution in the magnified image by scanning the patient initially with smaller data-sampling increments, possibly accompanied by a smaller aperture for the detector collimators. This approach yields improved resolution in the magnified image by accumulating data for a larger display matrix than is used in the nonmagnified image. Smaller apertures are not required with third-generation scanners since the beam width already is very narrow. In third-generation scanners, the spatial resolution is determined primarily by the data-sampling interval, and it can be improved by interlacing data obtained from opposite sides of the patient.

A second approach to magnified images with higher resolution involves scanning a region of interest that is smaller than the patient. The scanning is performed with smaller data-sampling increments than those normally employed. The region of interest is imaged over the

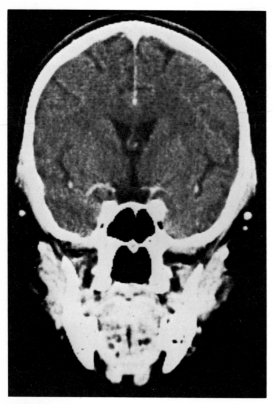

FIGURE 4-3. *Coronal image of interest reconstructed from measurements of x-ray transmission through several transaxial sections through the patient. (Courtesy of Medical Systems Division, General Electric Company.)*

entire display matrix so that each element of the display presents a magnified image of the corresponding volume of tissue. Limited region-of-interest (termed *limited-view*) scans are not possible with third-generation CT units.

Most CT units of recent vintage provide the capability of software manipulation of CT numbers so that coronal, sagittal, and oblique reconstructions can be displayed on the viewing console. These reconstructions are obtained by combining CT numbers along planes through adjacent sections. If the sections are relatively thick (10 mm or so), the resulting image is rather chunky and displeasing to the eye. Combining data from thinner sections provides a manipulated image that is more esthetic, but the image may be noisier, or the data accumulation time may be longer. For these reasons, sagittal, coronal, and oblique images usually are reconstructed over rather narrow regions of interest. A coronal image reconstructed from transaxial measurements of x-ray transmission is shown in Figure 4-3.

A variety of other options for image manipulation usually are available to the operator of a CT unit. For example, a "smoothing" operation may be available to diminish the visibility of image noise and thereby improve the visualization of low contrast structures in the image [4, 5]. Image smoothing may be accomplished at the time of image reconstruction, in which case the smoothing operation is termed a *preprocessing operation*. Alternatively, the smoothing process may be applied to the reconstructed data, an operation known as *postprocessed smoothing*.

Images also can be manipulated so that they display enhanced edges at boundaries between different structures. Edge-enhanced images sometimes yield improved visualization of small high-contrast objects. The edge-enhancement process also increases the disturbing effects of image noise, however, and edge-enhancement routines are used only rarely by most CT operators. Smoothed and edge-enhanced CT images are reproduced in Figure 4-4.

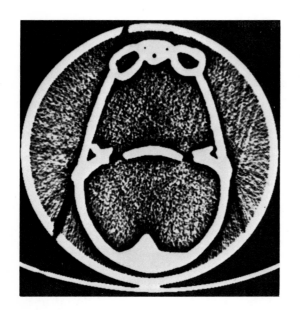 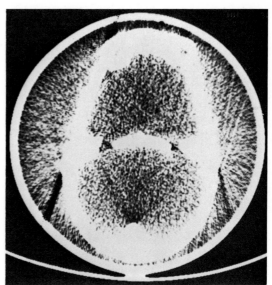

FIGURE 4-4.   *A test object imaged at constant window width and level but with "sharp"* (left) *and "smooth"* (right) *reconstruction algorithms.*

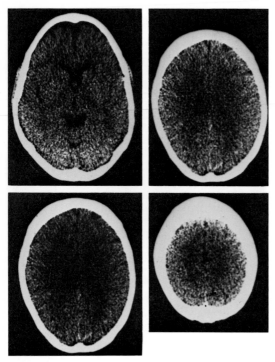

FIGURE 4-5. *Recording of four CT images on a single photographic film in a multiformat camera.*

Recent software developments for CT scanners have led to various additional techniques for image manipulation. For example, two images obtained with and without a contrast agent, or at different beam energies, can be subtracted to reveal anatomic details that are not visible in the original images. Temporal and energy-subtraction techniques in computed tomography are discussed in Chapter 13. In addition, sophisticated software routines are becoming available for beam-hardening corrections to the reconstructed image, for statistical analysis of CT numbers in a region of interest, and for determination of spatial and temporal changes in CT numbers, all of which may prove to have considerable clinical utility. Development of these types of software packages for image analysis represents one of the major areas of CT advancement anticipated for the near future. Some of these advancements are discussed in Chapter 13.

A variety of photographic methods are used to produce a permanent record of images on the viewing console. The use of Polaroid film is a common but expensive procedure, and the images are inconvenient to view and rather bulky to store. Also in widespread use are 70, 100, and 105 mm film formats. The perference today is for a multiformat camera, in which a selected number of images can be stored on one sheet of photographic film. Shown in Figure 4-5 are four images recorded on one sheet of 8- × 10-in. photographic film in a multiformat camera. To record a series of images in the multiformat camera, the film is moved to successive locations behind a lens system through which each of the images to be recorded is projected in sequence from the TV monitor. The film can be processed in a standard x-ray film processor, and the resultant images can be viewed and copied in the same manner as x-ray film. X-ray film is less expensive than Polaroid, but the cost of a multiformat camera is many times that of a Polaroid camera.

As an option (at extra cost), most CT scanners can be equipped with a high-speed printer that records the actual CT numbers constituting a CT image. A printer is especially useful for quality control of the CT scanner and for quantitative interpretation of the CT numbers comprising a CT image.

REFERENCES

1. Boyd, D., et al. A high-pressure xenon proportional chamber for x-ray laminographic reconstruction using fan-beam geometry. *IEEE Trans. Nucl. Sci.* 21:184, 1974.
2. Freundlich, D., and Zaklad, H. Detector Systems. Sec. II. Scintillation Crystal–Photomultiplier Tube Detectors. In T. H. Newton and D. G. Potts (eds.), *Radiology of the Skull and Brain: Technical Aspects of Computed Tomography.* St. Louis: Mosby, 1981. P. 4104.
3. Haque, P. Detector Systems. Sec. IV. Scintillation Crystal–Photodiode Array Detectors. In T. H. Newton and D. G. Potts (eds.), *Radiology of the Skull and Brain: Technical Aspects of Computed Tomography.* St. Louis: Mosby, 1981. P. 4127.
4. Hounsfield, G. N. Potential uses of more accurate CT absorption values by filtering. *Am. J. Roentgenol.* 131:103, 1978.
5. Joseph, P. M. Image noise and smoothing in computed tomography (CT) scanners. *Proceedings of the Society of Photo-Optical Instrumentation Engineers: Application of Optical Instrumentation in Medicine VI* 127:43, 1977.
6. Judy, P. F. The line-spread function and modulation transfer function of a computed tomographic scanner. *Med. Phys.* 3:233, 1976.
7. McCullough, E. D., and Payne, J. T. X-ray–transmission computed tomography. *Med. Phys.* 4:85, 1977.
8. Peschmann, K. Detector systems. Sec. III. Xenon Gas Ionization Detectors. In T. H. Newton and D. G. Potts (eds.), *Radiology of the Skull and Brain: Technical Aspects of Computed Tomography.* St. Louis: Mosby, 1981. P. 4112.
9. Zatz, L. M. General Overview of Computed Tomography Instrumentation. In T. H. Newton and D. G. Potts (eds.), *Radiology of the Skull and Brain: Technical Aspects of Computed Tomography.* St. Louis: Mosby, 1981. P. 4025.

5

Reconstruction of the Tomographic Image

In the completion of a computed tomographic (CT) scan across one section through a patient, thousands of measurements are obtained of the transmission of x rays through the patient. These measurements are obtained along many transmission "rays" through the patient at many different angular projections, or "views." From these transmission measurements, a matrix of CT numbers is computed for the cross-sectional plane through the patient. The CT numbers are related to linear attenuation coefficients and can be displayed as a gray-scale image. An explanation of various computational approaches to converting the transmission measurements into CT numbers is provided in this chapter. These computational approaches are inherently highly mathematical, and a full explanation requires a rather rigorous mathematical background. Only a conceptual explanation is offered here; more complete explanations are available in the literature [1–6].

Three mathematical methods have been employed for reconstruction of medical images from x-ray transmission data. These methods are (1) simple back-projection, (2) filtered back-projection, and (3) iterative reconstruction.

SIMPLE BACK-PROJECTION

Suppose that the transmission of x rays through a spherical object is measured along many rays from two views at right angles to each other. At each view, the measurements constitute a profile of x-ray transmission for a particular angular orientation. X-ray transmission profiles are shown in Figure 5-1.

After the x-ray transmission profiles have been obtained, the process of data accumulation can be reversed, to form a crude image of the sphere. The reversal process, known as *back-projection*, is easily implemented without sophis-

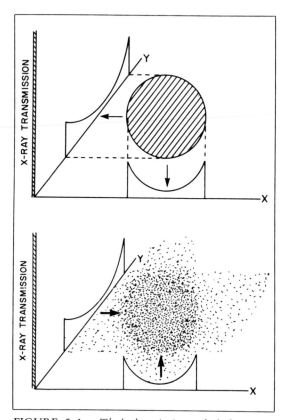

FIGURE 5-1. *The back-projection method of image reconstruction. Shown are two profiles of x-ray transmission through a spherical object. A crude image of the sphere* (bottom) *results from back-projecting the transmission profiles.*

ticated mathematics. For example, simple back-projection can be performed optically with photographic images obtained at a variety of angles. In the example in Figure 5-1, the image of the sphere would be improved if more profiles were obtained at different angles.

Simple back-projection techniques can be explained in another way. Suppose that a series of x-ray transmission measurements are made at different orientations across a single plane through the cube shown in Figure 5-2 (*top*), resulting in the x-ray transmission data noted on the axes. To initiate back-projection, each transmission ray is divided into ten parts. Along the x axis, each ray reveals either 20 or 40 percent transmission, corresponding to 80 and 60 percent attenuation, respectively. In simple back-projection, each part of the ray is assumed to contribute equally to the absorption. Hence, each part contributes 6 percent attenuation along the 40 percent transmission rays, and 8 percent attenuation along the 20 percent transmission rays along both the x and the y axes. In Figure 5-2 (*bottom*) these attenuation figures are added along a single plane in the cube to illustrate the effect of back-projecting the transmission data. In the cross-hatched area, projected attenuations of 8 percent per element from each axis add to form a total attenuation of 16 percent. In the diagonally hatched elements, a projected attenuation of 8 percent from one axis combines with an attenuation of 6 percent from the other axis to yield a total attenuation of 14 percent. The total attenuation is 12 percent in the clear elements. By shading the elements differently according to their relative attenuation values, a gray-scale reproduction is obtained of the plane through the cube across which the attenuation measurements were made. With more rays and views, the reproduction more nearly resembles the object.

A process similar to that depicted in Figure 5-2 could be used to provide a gray-scale display of a CT image. The image would be less than satis-

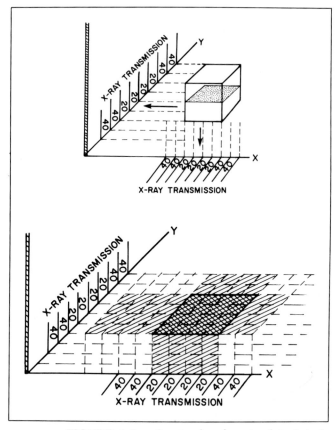

FIGURE 5-2.   *Conceptual mathematics of simple back-projection. Top: X-ray transmission across a single plane of the cube measured from two orientations at right angles to each other. The measurement plane is indicated by closely spaced dots. Bottom: The percent attenuation is divided equally among each of ten parts of each ray, and the attenuations are added in each intersecting element to yield values of 16 percent (8% + 8%) in each cross-hatched element, 14 percent (6% + 8%) in each diagonally hatched element, and 12 percent (6% + 6%) in each clear element.*

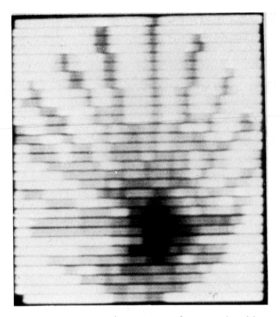

FIGURE 5-3. *Spoke pattern artifacts contributed by dense structures in images reconstructed by simple back-projection. (Reprinted from D. E. Kuhl, et al. Quantitative section scanning using orthogonal tangent correction.* J. Nucl. Med. *14:196, 1973. With permission.)*

factory, however, because the projected attenuations are averaged along the entire transmission ray and are not confined to the object of interest. For this reason, dense regions in the original object create a spoke pattern in the reconstructed image, as is shown in Figure 5-3. If many views of the object are used to create the image, the spoke pattern can be reduced but, concomitantly, a general blurring of the image occurs. These spoke-pattern artifacts and blurring processes have limited the usefulness of simple back-projection reconstruction techniques in clinical imaging.

FILTERED BACK-PROJECTION

To reduce spoke-pattern artifacts and blurring in back-projected images, the x-ray transmission data can be modified (filtered) before they are analyzed to form an image. The filtering process adds negative components to the back-projected data, so that the spokes are eliminated to a reasonable degree. By proper selection of the filtering function (or "deblurring function"), the blurring in the image is reduced, and the image resembles the object more closely.

The process of combining the projection data with a filter function is referred to as *convolving* the function with the data, and the technique is known as the *convolution method.* This method provides both speed and accuracy for image reconstruction, and it is the most widely used technique for image reconstruction in CT scanners available commercially. It has the further advantage that reconstruction of the image can proceed while x-ray transmission data are being collected. In this manner, the time between scanning and the availability of the reconstructed image can be reduced. Although there are variations in the detailed approach to filtered back-projection, a description of the distinction among these variations is beyond the scope of

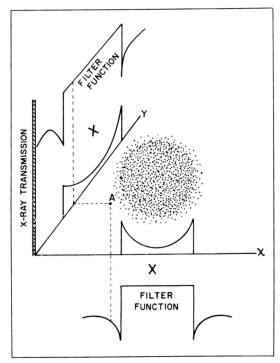

FIGURE 5-4. *X-ray transmission data in Figure 5-1 convolved with a filter function to improve the sharpness of the reconstructed image. The point A outside the object receives a positive contribution from the filter function on the y axis and a negative contribution from the filter function on the x axis.*

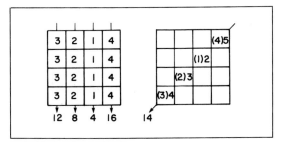

FIGURE 5-5. *Example of the iterative technique of image reconstruction for a 4 × 4 matrix of attenuation coefficients. A "first guess" of the coefficients is shown on the left, and an "improved guess" is shown on the right, after consideration of additional transmission data. (Reprinted from E. C. McCullough, and J. T. Payne, X-ray transmission computed tomography. Med. Phys. 4:85, 1977. With permission.)*

this text. The convolution method of image reconstruction is illustrated in Figure 5-4.

ITERATIVE RECONSTRUCTION

In the iterative reconstruction technique, values initially are assumed for the matrix of attenuation coefficients used to form the reconstruction image. As the transmission data are examined, inaccuracies in the assumed coefficients become evident, and corrections are made in the coefficients to achieve better agreement with the transmission data. This process is repeated many times in an iterative fashion, with the corrections becoming smaller and smaller until a satisfactory matrix of attenuation coefficients is obtained.

The iterative approach to image reconstruction is shown in Figure 5-5. On the left, a first guess of "attenuation data" is shown, with the data sum for each column compiled at the bottom of the diagram. For the next projection, a data sum of 14 was obtained for the transmission ray projected as a diagonal from the upper right to the bottom left. The value of 14 is greater than the expected value of 10 revealed by the first-guess attenuation data. The discrepancy of 4 is divided among the four elements along the diagonal so that each element is increased by 1 to yield the values outside the parentheses. These values become the new attenuation data, and the process is repeated in iterative fashion until the changes in attenuation data are minimal from one step to the next.

With iterative reconstruction techniques, essentially all the x-ray transmission data must be collected before the image can be reconstructed. Hence, image reconstruction times are longer with this approach than with the convolution method. These longer times were tolerable with earlier scanners because the data accumulation time was so long that a few seconds more or less for image reconstruction were not significant.

With the faster third- and fourth-generation scanners, image reconstruction time often limits the rate at which patients can be examined. Hence, iterative reconstruction techniques are not used with these scanners.

There are three basic versions of the iterative reconstruction technique: ILST (iterative least squares technique), SIRT (simultaneous iterative reconstruction technique), and ART (algebraic reconstruction technique). Distinction among these versions is beyond the scope of this text.

REFERENCES

1. Brooks, R. A., and Di Chiro, G. Beam hardening in x-ray reconstruction tomography. *Phys. Med. Biol.* 21:390, 1976.
2. Gordon, R., and Herman, G. T. Three-dimensional reconstruction from projections: A review of algorithms. *Int. Rev. Cytol.* 38:111, 1974.
3. Herman, G. T. Principles of Reconstruction Algorithms. Sec. II. Advanced Principles of Reconstruction Algorithms. In T. H. Newton and D. G. Potts (eds.), *Radiology of the Skull and Brain: Technical Aspects of Computed Tomography.* St. Louis: Mosby, 1981. P. 3888.
4. Kak, A. C. Computerized tomography with x-ray, emission, and ultrasound sources. *Proc. IEEE* 67:1245, 1979.
5. Macovski, A. Principles of Reconstruction Algorithms. Sec. I. Basic Concepts of Reconstruction Algorithms. In T. H. Newton and D. G. Potts (eds.), *Radiology of the Skull and Brain: Technical Aspects of Computed Tomography.* St. Louis: Mosby, 1981. P. 3877.
6. Ramachandran, G. N., and Lakshminarayanan, A. V. Three-dimensional reconstruction from radiographs and electron micrographs: Application of convolutions instead of Fourier transforms. *Proc. Natl. Acad. Sci.* 68:2236, 1971.

6

Data Acquisition and Computer Systems in Computed Tomography

The computer is the heart of any computed tomographic (CT) scanner, for without the "number-crunching" capability of modern digital computers, the reconstruction of clinical images from measurements of x-ray transmission would be impractical, if not impossible. In many ways, a modern CT scanner can be characterized as a digital computer with an x-ray tube and a few radiation detectors attached to one end and a viewing device for the presentation of images attached to the other end (Figure 6-1). CT could not have developed much earlier than the 1970s because it relies on fast and inexpensive minicomputers dedicated to tasks such as image reconstruction. These minicomputers were developed in the late 1960s.

Although computers were used in nuclear medicine in the 1960s, their introduction into the general field of radiologic imaging dates from the implementation of computed tomography in 1972. This introduction probably will eventually be recognized as a turning point in the evolution of diagnostic radiology. Even today, major changes are becoming apparent in radiology as computers become an essential part of state-of-the-art imaging processes such as real-time ultrasound, digital radiography, emission tomography, and nuclear magnetic resonance. In all likelihood, computers will be as essential to the radiologist of the future as x-ray tubes are to the radiologist of today. For this reason, persons interested in the processes of forming and interpreting radiologic images should understand at least the rudiments of computer terminology and operation.

The term *computer* is a general expression encompassing a number of specific components of a computed tomographic unit. A better term than computer for these components is *data pro-*

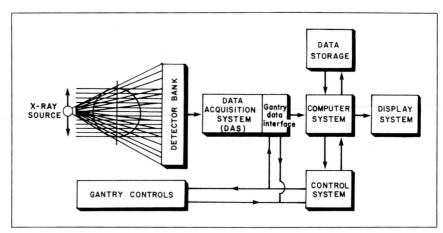

FIGURE 6-1. *Major components of a CT unit. (Reprinted from B. M. Gordon, Data Acquisition Systems. In T. H. Newton and D. G. Potts {eds.}*, Radiology of the Skull and Brain: Technical Aspects of Computed Tomography. *St. Louis: Mosby, 1981. With permission.)*

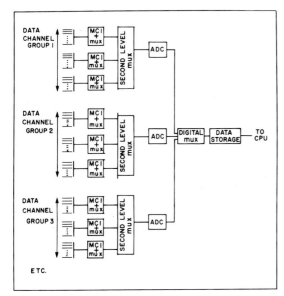

FIGURE 6-2.   *Diagram of a typical data acquisition system. MCI = multichannel integrator; MUX = multiplexer; ADC = analog digital converter.*

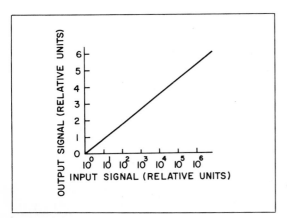

FIGURE 6-3.   *Relationship of output to input signal in a logarithmic amplifier.*

cessing system, with the components identified as the data acquisition system, the central processing unit, the memory, input-output devices, and peripherals. Each of these components is discussed in this chapter and Chapter 7.

DATA ACQUISITION SYSTEM

The data acquisition system (DAS) provides an interface between the x-ray portion of a CT scanner and the central processing unit that uses measurements of x-ray transmission to reconstruct an image. The DAS accepts electrical signals from the radiation detectors, converts these signals into a digital format suitable for computer processing, and transmits the converted signals to the central processing unit. The DAS is probably the most sophisticated and expensive part of a CT unit, and problems occurring in the DAS can have disastrous consequences on the quality of the reconstructed image.

Shown in Figure 6-2 are the major components of a data acquisition system used in a typical CT unit. Some of these components are required and others are optional, depending on the configuration of the CT unit and the data format required by the central processing unit.

Electrical signals from the radiation detectors may vary in magnitude by factors as large as 10 [5]. These signals must be amplified and measured with high accuracy, and logarithmic amplifiers often satisfy these criteria best. As is shown in Figure 6-3, logarithmic amplifiers furnish an output signal that is proportional to the logarithm of the input signal. In this manner, the range of output signals is significantly compressed compared to the range of incoming signals. Logarithmic amplifiers require periodic calibration to ensure that the amplification characteristics do not drift with time or environmental conditions [1].

After logarithmic amplification, signals from the detectors are collected by *integration circuits.* The function of an integration circuit is to pro-

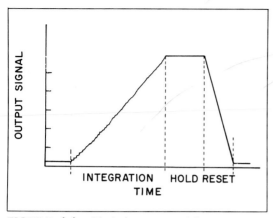

FIGURE 6-4. *Typical output signal from an integration circuit.*

vide an output signal that represents the sum of all the input signals received over a specified period of time. In a CT unit with a pulsed x-ray beam, for example, the integration circuit yields an output voltage proportional to the sum of the input signals received during a single x-ray pulse. This output voltage is retained by the integration circuit until it can be transferred to the next stage in the data acquisition system. That is, there is a hold period for the integrated signal while it awaits transfer. After the hold period, the integration circuit is reset, to be ready to receive signals during the next x-ray pulse. The production of an output signal in an integration circuit is depicted in Figure 6-4.

Signals stored in the integration circuits are transferred to a time-shared *analog-digital converter* (ADC) for conversion into digital format. The signals from a bank of integration circuits are transferred one at a time to a common ADC by use of a multiplexer. Essentially, a *multiplexer* is a group of electronic switches with control circuits that turn the switches on and off.

The conversion of electrical signals from analog to digital format occurs in the analog-digital converter. The input to an ADC is usually a voltage signal, and the output is a numeric code representing the magnitude of the voltage signal. The accuracy of the conversion from analog to digital format depends in part on how well the range of analog signals can be separated into different numeric codes. No matter how fine the conversion of analog to digital signals is, however, some error always occurs as analog signals are "rounded" up or down to the nearest numeric code. This error is termed *quantization noise* or *round-off error* [2].

In *linear ADCs,* the output numeric code varies linearly with the magnitude of the input signal. Linear ADCs often are limited in their response to the wide range of input signals provided in many CT units. This limitation can be alleviated by using either a linear floating-point ADC or a logarithmic ADC.

In a linear floating-point ADC, the input signal is amplified automatically by a predetermined amount (e.g., 1, 8, or 64) depending on whether the size of the input signal is large, intermediate, or small. In this manner, input signals are scaled automatically to fall within the response range of the ADC. In a *logarithmic ADC*, the output numeric code is proportional to the logarithm of the ratio of a reference signal to the signal being measured.

After conversion by the ADCs, the digital signals are multiplexed into the central processing unit of the data processing system (Figure 6-2). The digital multiplexing operation may include temporary storage of the data for accessing by the processing section at a later time.

CENTRAL PROCESSING UNIT

The central processing unit (CPU) is the section of the data processing system in which all arithmetic operations occur. These operations are governed by instructions such as "add," "subtract," "branch," and others that are stored in computer memory and accessed by the CPU whenever needed. A sequence of instructions that yields a specific result is termed a *program,* and a portion of this sequence (e.g., an arithmetic operation such as taking the square root) that can be implemented by a single instruction is termed a *subroutine*. Increasingly, subroutines are being replaced by microprogrammed architectures that are much faster than subroutines in performing arithmetic operations.

The introduction of *integrated circuit chips* in the 1970s has resulted in the rapid evolution of faster and more powerful CPUs that are less expensive to purchase and easier to program and use. This evolution has led to microprocessors, minicomputers, and array processors, which are now finding application in virtually all areas of diagnostic imaging.

Array processors are integrated circuits designed to perform certain mathematical operations on data arranged in the form of arrays. With this approach, massive amounts of data can be handled very efficiently. Array processors commonly are used in signal-processing applications such as computed tomography.

MEMORY

The *memory* is that part of a data processing system in which data, computational results, instructions, and other details, are stored when they are not being used by the CPU. These quantities can be transferred almost instantaneously between the memory and the CPU. Two types of memory are commonly available— magnetic core memories and semiconductor memories [3].

All computer operations can be resolved into choices between two alternatives, such as yes/ no, on/off, or 0/1. The choice of one of two alternatives is a *bit* (*bi*nary digi*t*) of information. For example, suppose the number 43 is to be stored in computer memory. The number is translated into binary format as 0 or 1 times successive powers of 2; that is, 43 is translated as $(1 \times 2^5) + (0 \times 2^4) + (1 \times 2^3) + (0 \times 2^2) + (1 \times 2^1) + (1 \times 2^0)$ and expressed as 101011.

A *magnetic core memory* contains many tiny rings of ferromagnetic material, with one ring for each bit of core memory. An electrical pulse transmitted through a wire centered in each ring can magnetize the ring either clockwise or counterclockwise, to represent either unity or zero. When the memory is "read" (i.e., when data or instructions are taken from the memory), the magnetization of the rings is destroyed and must be restored by remagnetization. A memory with remagnetization capability is said to be "nonvolatile," because the contents of the memory are preserved when power to the data processing system is suspended.

A semiconductor memory uses integrated circuit chips (IC chips) in place of ferromagnetic

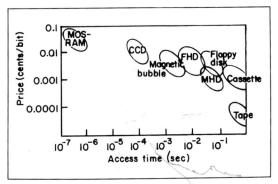

FIGURE 6-5. *Cost per bit versus access time for various types of memory systems. (Reprinted from A. J. Grant, J. J. Morrissey, and R. B. Diederich, Computers in Computed Tomography. In T. H. Newton and D. G. Potts {eds.}, Radiology of the Skull and Brain: Technical Aspects of Computed Tomography. St. Louis: Mosby, 1981. With permission.)*

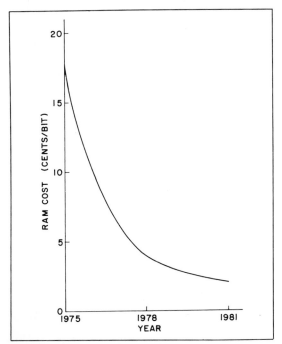

FIGURE 6-6. *Reductions in cost per bit in random access memories over the past few years. (Plotted from data in G. W. Schultz, Computed Tomograpy Displays. In T. H. Newton and D. G. Potts {eds.}, Radiology of the Skull and Brain: Technical Aspects of Computed Tomography. St. Louis: Mosby, 1981. With permission.)*

rings and is faster and less expensive than a magnetic core memory. Some of the newer types of semiconductor memories—e.g., charge-coupled devices (CCD), magnetic bubbles, and metal oxide semiconductor random access memories (MOS-RAM)—are compared in Figure 6-5 to more conventional memory systems such as fixed (FHD) and moving (MHD) head disks. Dramatic reductions in the cost per bit of information stored in memory have been realized in the last few years, as shown in Figure 6-6. With most semiconductor memories, the content of the memory is destroyed if power to the system is suspended.

In computer terminology, a *bit* is a unit of information that can be described by the notation 1 or 0 as represented, for example, by the state of magnetization of a single ferromagnetic ring in a magnetic-core memory. Eight bits constitute a *byte* and provide a sufficiently large data field to describe any alphabetic character or decimal digit. The size of a computer memory is described in units of either bytes or words. Memories in units of *kilobytes* (1,000 bytes) or *megabytes* (1 million bytes) are common. Sometimes memory sizes are described in units of words, where a *word* is the smallest data field that can describe an instruction. Memories of 16- and 32-bit words are commonplace.

INPUT/OUTPUT DEVICES
The input/output (I/O) section of a data processing system is the method of communication of the system with the external world. With this section, data can be transmitted between the processing system and external instruments such as electromechanical equipment, display devices such as video terminals and line printers, and data-storage mechanisms such as magnetic-disk and tape drives. The transmission may occur over telephone lines, through cables, or by modulation of light waves, microwaves, or other

electromagnetic radiations. Two types of data transfer through I/O devices generally are available. These types are programmed I/O and data channel I/O.

Programmed I/O is used predominantly when data are transferred between the CPU and relatively slow devices such as floppy disks, magnetic tape, and low-speed printers. The data-transfer process is controlled by a subroutine stored either in main memory or, possibly, on a disk. Programmed I/O is not suitable for data transfer with high-speed devices such as disks because the I/O section cannot process the data rapidly enough. With a *data channel*, blocks of data can be transferred in and out of main memory directly, without passing through the CPU. Hence, data transmission is much more rapid with a data channel than with programmed I/O.

PERIPHERALS

In a data processing system, *peripherals* are devices used for storage and display of data generated by the system. These devices include disks, tapes, array processors and various data-display units such as printers, video terminals, and operating consoles. These devices are discussed in Chapter 7.

LANGUAGES

The CPU of a data processing system responds to instructions written in *assembly* or *machine* language. The instructions are written in a numeric code employing 1s and 0s and are lengthy and difficult to prepare. For this reason, almost all data processing systems are equipped with *compilers* for translation into assembly language of a series of comments written in a higher-level computer language.

Various higher level languages exist, each of which requires a compiler designed for a specific data processing system. Programming codes such as FORTRAN, COBOL, and PL/1 are examples of higher-level languages that are much easier to understand and use when compared to an assembly language. However, assembly language programs usually use the data processing system more efficiently.

Recently, the major advances in CT technology have been more in software developments than in hardware. Dynamic scanning, statistical evaluations of groups of CT data, image manipulation, and more rapid reconstruction times are examples of software improvements; further advances may be expected in the near future.

REFERENCES

1. Gordon, B. M. Data Acquisition Systems. In T. H. Newton and D. G. Potts (eds.), *Radiology of the Skull and Brain: Technical Aspects of Computed Tomography.* St. Louis: Mosby, 1981. P. 4133.
2. Gordon, B. M. Linear electronic analog-digital conversion architectures, their origins, parameters, limitations, and applications. IEEE *Trans. Circ. Syst.* CAS-25:391, 1978.
3. Grant, A. J., Morrissey, J. J., and Diederich, R. B. Computers in Computed Tomography. In T. H. Newton and D. G. Potts (eds.), *Radiology of the Skull and Brain: Technical Aspects of Computed Tomography.* St. Louis: Mosby, 1981. P. 4159.

7 Data Display and Recording

Data generated by a computed tomographic (CT) unit are presented in the form of CT numbers that are related directly to linear attenuation coefficients. To be clinically useful, these data must be transformed into a visual image, in which various regions of anatomy are depicted as different shades of gray (or as different colors). This transformation is the function of the *visual display system,* and the heart of the display system is a cathode ray tube (CRT) operated as a video terminal.

A CRT consists of an electron gun that directs a beam of electrons in a scanning pattern across the back surface of a fluorescent screen. By changing the intensity of the electron beam, the amount of light released from each part of the screen is varied to produce a gray-scale image of the value of CT numbers across a tissue section through the patient. The fluorescent material in the CRT screen has a low persistence (i.e., the fluorescence decays rapidly), so that a crisp and clear image is obtained. However, the image must be recreated (i.e., "refreshed") many times each second to yield an image of constant brightness on the fluorescent screen. If the refresh rate is too low, the image will appear to flicker and will cause distraction and eye fatigue in the viewer.

Refresh rates of 60 images per second typically are employed in video displays used with CT units in the United States. (The refresh rate must be identical to, or a multiple of, the frequency of fluorescent ambient light; otherwise there will be a beat frequency, equal to the difference in the frequencies of the refresh rate and the fluorescent light, that causes the image to flicker.) To refresh the image, the electron beam must rescan the entire fluorescent screen once every $\frac{1}{60}$ second. In ordinary television, each rescan is interlaced with the preceding electron beam scan so that a complete image (i.e., a single television frame) of interlaced scan lines is

Table 7-1. *Characteristics of Broadcast Television and CT Video Displays*

Value	CT	Television
Total number of elements per line	395	395
Total number of visible elements per line	320	320
Total number of lines	525	525
Total number of visible lines	480	480
Line frequency (sec^{-1})	31,500	15,750
Field frequency	—	60
Frame frequency	60	30
Time for one complete line (μsec)	31.8	63.5
Time for one element (ηsec)	80.5	161
Effective element frequency (MHz)	12.44	6.22

Source: Modified from Schultz, G. W. Computed Tomography Displays. In T. H. Newton and D. G. Potts (eds.), *Radiology of the Skull and Brain: Technical Aspects of Computed Tomography*. St. Louis: Mosby, 1981. P. 4173. With permission.

created every $\frac{1}{30}$ second [2]. Video display systems do not use an interlaced format; instead, a complete image or television frame is created by a single raster scan every $\frac{1}{60}$ second. In this approach, data are transmitted and displayed at twice the frequency of ordinary television, and faster and more costly electronics are required. Broadcast television and CT video displays are compared in Table 7-1.

As can be seen from Table 7-1, the number of picture elements per second that are displayed and refreshed in a CT image on a video display is

Number of elements per second = (395 elements per line) (525 lines per frame) (60 frames per second) = 12.44 million

To provide a separate shade of gray for each picture element, the intensity of the electron beam must change at this frequency. That is, CT numbers that influence the intensity of the electron beam must be extracted from computer memory at a frequency of 12.44 MHz. With consideration of lines and elements that are not displayed, this frequency yields a maximum time per element of 80.5 ηsec (Table 7-1). The portion of computer memory where the CT numbers are stored is termed the *refresh memory* because the numbers are read out repeatedly and sequentially at very high rates to refresh the displayed image. Each location (*address*) in this refresh memory corresponds to a single set of spatial coordinates on the video display screen, and the CT number stored at that location determines the gray-scale level of the image at that set of coordinates. Display systems operated in this fashion are termed *raster scan bit*-per-element display systems [3].

CT numbers stored in the refresh memory may range from $-1,000$ to $1,000$ (or higher). When these numbers are displayed in a visual image, each of the numbers theoretically should be represented as a different shade of gray. However, the average human eye cannot distinguish more than 16 to 20 shades of gray. Although a physician trained in viewing gray-scale images may be able to differentiate more shades of gray, his or her talent certainly does not extend beyond perhaps 64 gray levels. Even with this extended capability, 2,000/64 (or about 30 CT numbers) would be associated with each perceived gray level. This degree of clumping of CT numbers is far too coarse to permit visual distinction of tissues that differ slightly in CT number.

To improve the visualization of tissues with slight differences in CT values, one or more display windows with selectable position and width are provided on CT units. The position of the window on the scale of CT numbers is determined with a window level control that resembles the brightness control on a standard television set. The window width control determines the range of CT values that is displayed as black to white in the image. This control resembles the contrast control on a standard television set. With the window level and width controls, any range of CT numbers may be displayed as black to white in the image presented on the display device.

Display devices provide additional features that are useful in viewing CT images. For example, images can be magnified by replacing each pixel in a region by a sequence of perhaps four pixels with the same CT value. The replacement provides $2 \times$ magnification for a quarter of the image originally projected on the viewing screen. In many CT units, a light pen can be used to define a region of interest (ROI) in the image, and the arithmetic mean and standard deviation of the CT numbers within the ROI can be computed. With this capability, comparative evaluations of mean CT numbers between different regions can be performed, and changes in mean CT numbers within a ROI can be analyzed as a function of time to provide a CT index of dynamic processes in the body. In addition, CT images usually can be annotated with character information, and graphics software can be used to display graphic information. In most CT units, successive CT sections can be integrated to provide coronal and sagittal images, usually with rather poor spatial resolution unless very thin transaxial sections are taken close together.

One innovative feature of some display units is introduction of a nonlinear relationship between CT numbers and the gray-scale display of these numbers. This relationship compensates for the nonlinear response of the photographic system or the human eye to a gray-scale image [1, 4]. That is, the gray-scale image is skewed purposely to make it appear linear to the observer.

INTERACTIVE PERIPHERALS

Interactive peripherals are one-way communication devices that give the operator some control over the display system. Among these peripherals are keyboards, joysticks, trackballs, light pens, potentiometers, and tablets.

A *keyboard* resembles a scaled-down version of a typewriter keyboard. Some keyboards are essentially numbers only, while others are alphanumeric keyboards, which provide both numbers and letters. Keyboards are a series of electronic switches that are closed by depressing a key. They are used routinely for operations such as control of the scanning process, storage and retrieval of images, and annotation of images.

Joysticks are combinations of potentiometers or electronic switches used to control the movement of a cursor on the display screen. A *cursor* is a small, bright cross hair or blinking dot that can be superimposed on the video image to identify pixels, outline regions of interest, or draw lines on the display. The joystick can move the cursor at constant speed or at a speed that varies with displacement of the joystick from its equilibrium position.

Cursors also can be controlled with a *trackball mechanism* consisting of a plastic ball whose rotational orientation is detected by an array of phototransistor sensors that specify the coordinates $\pm$ x and $\pm$ y. The speed of cursor movement is determined by the rate of rotation of the trackball. Trackballs are more sensitive than joysticks and are preferred by some users because they provide a finer degree of control over movement of the cursor.

Light pens allow the operator to work directly on the fluorescent screen of the video display without having to rely on hand-eye coordination between cursor position and movement of a joystick or trackball. The light pen contains a light-sensing device that detects the electron beam as it scans across the inner surface of the screen. The location of the light pen on the screen is identified by the coordinates of the electron beam when a signal is generated in the light pen. Light pens sometimes fail to perform properly in dark regions of the image where insufficient light is present to generate a signal in the light pen.

A *tablet* is a surface that detects the position of a stylus held against it by the operator. The surface is essentially a grid of x-y coordinates that is correlated with the coordinates of the screen of the video display device. As the stylus is moved across the tablet, a cursor on the display screen visibly follows the movement. The method of detection of the position of the stylus on the tablet varies from one tablet to another.

IMAGE RECORDING
Recording on Film

CT images can be photographed directly on either Polaroid or conventional photographic film. Polaroid prints are positive images that are convenient to produce and store, but they are expensive and difficult to copy. Conventional film must be transilluminated for viewing and can be processed in an automatic film processor. With a multiformat camera, many images can be recorded on a single sheet of film. Either Polaroid or conventional film is capable of recording all the information in the image presented on the video display unit. However, the photographic image is not always as esthetically pleasing as the video image, because the gray-scale presentation is affected by the photographic process, and television raster lines are more apparent in the photographic image.

Disk Storage

Because CT presents data in digital form, the most convenient method of intermediate data storage usually is the *magnetic disk*. In this form of data storage, a ferromagnetic material is coated on a support base, which may be rigid (in a conventional disk) or flexible (in a floppy disk). The disk is used with one or more *read-write heads,* which induce and read patterns of magnetism on the disk. The disk is rotated at high speed, with the heads almost, but not quite, touching the magnetic surface of the disk. Although read-write heads may be either moving-head or fixed-head types, the moving-head type is used almost universally in computed tomography. In large disks, a stack of up to 19 magnetic surfaces (*platters*) is available for data recording. Large disks can store up to 300 million eight-bit bytes (300 megabytes) of information. With data packing, a single CT image requires about 0.2 megabyte of storage.

Floppy disks provide a flexible recording surface and offer a convenient and inexpensive method of data storage. With a floppy disk, the read-write heads actually contact the recording surface, and the resulting abrasion affects the lifetime of the disk. This disadvantage usually is offset by the low cost and convenience of floppy disks.

For long-term storage of CT data, magnetic tape is almost always the preferred medium. *Magnetic tape* is similar to a magnetic disk except that the data are recorded linearly rather than in circular tracks. Magnetic tape contains multiple tracks (e.g., eight tracks) for data recording plus a single track, termed a *parity track,* for the verification of recorded data.

To retrieve data from magnetic tape, the tape must be read serially. Consequently, considerable time may be required to locate a record on magnetic tape, and use of this medium in CT is confined primarily to long-term storage of data.

Nonphotographic Storage

Different nonphotographic methods for data storage in computed tomography are compared in Table 7-2.

Table 7-2.   *Characteristics of Nonphotographic Storage Media in Computed Tomography*

Storage Medium	Cost (cents/bit)	Transfer Rate (words/sec)	Access Time
Magnetic core or semiconductor RAM	0.1–0.5	NA	1 sec
Magnetic disk	10^{-4}	$1–5 \times 10^5$	1–2 sec
Floppy disk	10^{-4}	$1–5 \times 10^4$	2–10 sec
Magnetic tape	2×10^{-5}	$\geq 10^3$	1 sec–5 min (serial access)

RAM = random access memory; NA = not available.

REFERENCES

1. Hall, C. F., and Hall, E. I. A nonlinear model for the spatial characteristics of the human visual system. *IEEE Trans. Syst. Mon. and Cybern. SMC* 7:161, 1977.

2. Hendee, W. R. *Medical Radiation Physics: Roentgenology, Nuclear Medicine, and Ultrasound* (2nd ed.). Chicago: Year Book, 1979. P. 331.

3. Schultz, G. W. Computed Tomography Displays. In T. H. Newton and D. G. Potts (eds.), *Radiology of the Skull and Brain: Technical Aspects of Computed Tomography*. St. Louis: Mosby, 1981. P. 4173.

4. Schwenker, R. P. Film Selection for Computed Tomography and Ultrasound Video Imaging. In A. G. Haus (ed.), *The Physics of Medical Imaging: Recording System Measurements and Techniques*. New York: American Institute of Physics, 1979. P. 381.

8 Performance Evaluation and Radiation Dose in Computed Tomography

A computed tomographic unit is a complex imaging instrument that requires careful evaluation of its performance before purchase, at the time of installation, and at frequent intervals after its introduction into clinical use. In addition, computed tomography (CT) delivers significant amounts of radiation to patients, and therefore techniques are needed to measure the radiation dose accompanying typical examination techniques.

Like all other radiologic images, those furnished by a CT unit exhibit features that should be evaluated as part of any protocol to assess the performance of the unit. These image features are (1) spatial resolution, (2) contrast resolution, (3) image noise, and (4) image distortion and artifacts. Each of these features is discussed at length in Chapters 9 and 10. In this chapter, concise definitions of the features are followed by a description of methods to evaluate them.

SPATIAL RESOLUTION

The *spatial resolution* of a CT unit is its ability to portray small structures that are separated only slightly in the object. Measurements of spatial resolution should be conducted in the absence of image noise; also, they usually are performed with test objects of high contrast. Often, the spatial resolution is determined with a test object containing small holes or pins separated by varying distances. The spatial resolution is described as the minimum distance between the holes or pins in the object that can be resolved in the image. This method is the most common approach to measurement of spatial resolution in a CT unit. Most CT units provide spatial resolution in the range of 1 to 2 mm, and some newer units demonstrate spatial resolution of less than

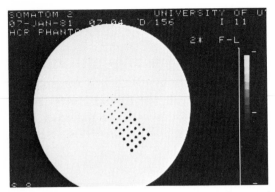

FIGURE 8-1. *Image of a high-contrast test object used to evaluate the spatial resolution of a CT unit.*

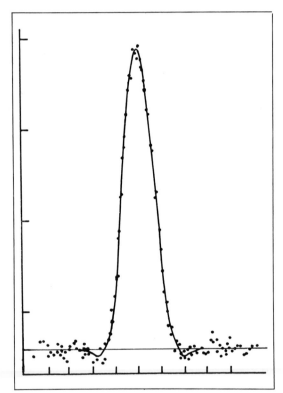

FIGURE 8-2. *Line-spread function for a representative CT unit. (From M. Bergstrom, Performance Evaluation of Scanners. In T. H. Newton and D. G. Potts {eds.}, Radiology of the Skull and Brain: Technical Aspects of Computed Tomography. St. Louis: Mosby, 1981. P. 4212. With permission.)*

1 mm. Because measurement of spatial resolution is influenced by the window width of the display unit, a width should be selected that is comparable to that used clinically. Figure 8-1 is an image of a plastic test object containing low-density pins from which an assessment of spatial resolution can be made.

An alternative approach to the measurement of spatial resolution involves determination of the degree of image blurring for a solitary line-shaped structure in the object. The degree of blurring is described as the *line-spread function* (Figure 8-2). The blurring exhibited by the line spread function often is described as the *full width at half maximum* (FWHM), defined as the fractional width of the line-spread function at half its maximum height. In Figure 8-2, for example, the FWHM is

$$\text{FWHM} = \frac{233 - 227}{230} \times 100 = 2.6\%$$

A higher value of the FWHM implies poorer spatial resolution.

From the line-spread function, a third measure of spatial resolution can be derived. This measure is termed the *modulation transfer function* (MTF), which essentially is a description of how sinusoidal fluctuations in x-ray transmission through the object are reproduced in the image (Figure 8-3). The maximum value of the MTF is unity, which indicates that sinusoidal fluctuations in x-ray transmission through the object are reproduced exactly in the image. An MTF value less than unity implies some loss of spatial resolution, and a value less than about 0.1 indicates that the image does not reveal fluctuations in x-ray intensity through the object. An MTF value of about 0.1 often is referred to as the *cutoff frequency*. The abscissa (x axis) of the MTF curve is denoted as spatial frequency and essentially is an indication of the spatial separation required for fluctuations in x-ray intensity in the object to be portrayed faithfully in the image.

Spatial resolution often varies markedly over

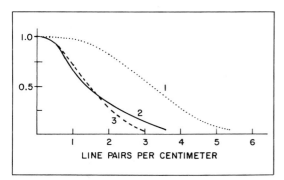

FIGURE 8-3.   *Modulation transfer functions computed for three CT units of relatively recent vintage.*

the image, and, consequently, measurements of spatial resolution should be obtained at a variety of positions within the field of view of the CT unit. In addition, comparative measurements of spatial resolution over time provide a quality control index of the performance reproducibility of the CT unit. Spatial resolution measurements are an integral part of the quality control program for a CT unit.

CONTRAST RESOLUTION

The term *contrast resolution* describes the ability of an x-ray imaging system to reveal subtle differences in the transmission of x rays through the object. Contrast resolution is an important property of CT images, because one of the principal advantages of CT is its ability to portray structures that differ only slightly from their surroundings in the transmission of x rays.

Contrast resolution can be evaluated subjectively with the use of images of a *test phantom* that contains structures differing only slightly from their surroundings in the transmission of x rays. For example, a plastic phantom with small depressions drilled to different depths can serve as a contrast-resolution phantom. Alternatively, holes drilled through a plastic phantom and filled with a solution that differs in its transmission characteristics slightly from the surrounding plastic can be used to evaluate contrast resolution. Figure 8-4 is an image from a contrast-resolution phantom.

Measurements of the contrast scale can be compared as a quantitative index of the low-contrast performance of a CT unit on a day-by-day basis. The *contrast scale* is computed as

$$\text{Contrast scale} = \frac{\mu_\rho - \mu_w}{(CT)_\rho - (CT)_w}$$

where μ_ρ and $(CT)_\rho$ refer to the linear attenuation coefficient and CT number for a selected plastic, and μ_w and $(CT)_w$ refer to the linear attenuation coefficient and CT number for wa-

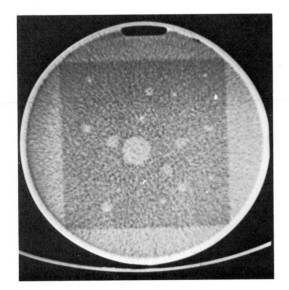 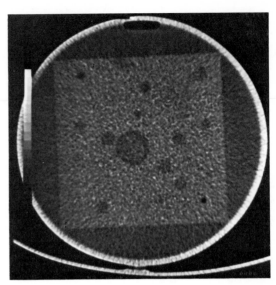

FIGURE 8-4. *Images of a contrast resolution phantom containing holes filled with solutions that are* (left) *slightly more dense and* (right) *slightly less dense than the surrounding plastic.*

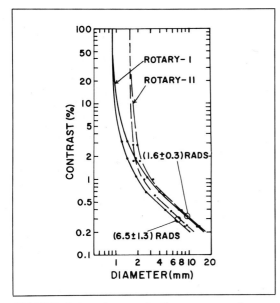

FIGURE 8-5.   *Contrast detail curves measured at two dose levels for two third generation CT units. (From G. Cohen and F. A. DiBianca, The use of contrast-detail-dose evaluation of image quality in a computed tomographic scanner. J. Comput. Assist. Tomogr. 3:189, 1979. With permission.)*

ter. For example, if the CT number difference is 122 HU (Hounsfield units) between Lucite and water, and the difference in linear attenuation coefficients is 0.024 cm^{-1} between the same materials, the contrast scale is

$$\text{Contrast scale} = \frac{0.024 \text{ cm}^{-1}}{122} = 0.00020 \text{ cm}^{-1}$$

per CT unit

This value corresponds approximately to a change of 100 in the CT value expressed in Hounsfield units for a 2 percent shift in the linear attenuation coefficient relative to water. In most CT units, the contrast scale varies somewhat with x-ray energy, so quality control measurements of the contrast scale always should be repeated at the same kilovolt peak (kVp) setting. For full characterization of this parameter, it should be measured at each kVp setting used clinically.

A more complete description of contrast resolution is furnished by a *contrast-detail (C-D) curve* [5]. A C-D curve is obtained with a phantom that contains structures of various sizes that differ slightly in x-ray transmission from the surrounding homogeneous medium. The contrast between a cylinder and the surrounding medium is expressed as the difference in CT number between the two materials, and a C-D curve is obtained when the CT-number differences for various materials are plotted against the size of the structures (Figure 8-5). C-D curves are useful in assessing the ability of a CT unit to discriminate small, low-contrast objects; however, they can yield misleading results under circumstances in which CT units with different x-ray beams are being compared [9]. Moreover, C-D curves vary with the level of noise present in the image and consequently are usually determined under relatively noise-free conditions.

Contrast resolution depends on the spectral distribution of x rays in the x-ray beam furnished by a CT unit. As a relatively coarse indi-

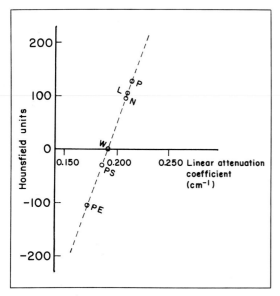

FIGURE 8-6. *A linear relationship is obtained when measured CT numbers are plotted against the linear attenuation coefficient of various materials for a photon energy of 73 keV. Hence, the effective photon energy is 73 keV. PE = polyethylene; PS = polystyrene; W = water; N = nylon; L = Lexan; and P = Perspex. (From M. Bergstrom, Performance Evaluation of Scanners. In T. H. Newton and D. G. Potts {eds.}, Radiology of the Skull and Brain: Technical Aspects of Computed Tomography. St. Louis: Mosby, 1981. P. 4212. With permission.)*

cation of the spectral distribution, the effective keV of the x-ray beam sometimes is described, in which keV (kiloelectron volt) is a unit of energy equal to the kinetic energy imparted to an electron accelerated through a potential difference of 1 volt. The *effective keV* is the energy of x rays in a monoenergetic beam that would be transmitted through a patient or test object in exactly the way the actual beam is transmitted. For a CT unit, the effective energy is identified by determining the x-ray energy at which the measured CT numbers are related linearly to known values of the linear attenuation coefficient for a variety of substances [12, 16]. Since the attenuation coefficient varies with energy, several energies usually must be assumed for the x-ray beam, and the one that yields a linear plot of CT number versus attenuation coefficient is taken as the effective energy (Figure 8-6). From a graph like that in Figure 8-6, the attenuation coefficient can be determined for any CT number measured with the CT unit, provided that the spectral distribution of the x-ray beam does not change [13]. The shape of the curve in Figure 8-6 also yields the contrast scale for the CT unit. At the extreme ends of the CT-number versus attenuation curve, some nonlinearity is encountered with most CT units.

The accuracy of CT numbers refers to the agreement between measured CT numbers and the values predicted from a curve like that in Figure 8-6. Factors that affect the accuracy of CT numbers include beam hardening [3], statistical imprecision related to image noise, and the size and shape of the object, as described in Chapters 9 and 10. The latter influences cause the CT numbers of specific tissues to vary with the size of the patient and the amount of bone present in the tissue section scanned, and is particularly troublesome when CT numbers of brain tissue are used as a quantitative index of pathology [6]. Methods to assess the effect of patient size and other factors on the CT numbers of specific tissues are described in the literature [2].

Spatial uniformity refers to the ability of a CT unit to yield the same CT number irrespective of the position of a structure within an otherwise homogeneous object. The major cause of spatial nonuniformity is beam hardening, and the degree of spatial uniformity achieved by a CT unit depends on the size and shape of the object scanned as well as the presence of high density objects such as bone. Spatial uniformity often is described by the maximum deviation of CT numbers from the mean CT number for a region of interest. Spatial uniformity also is affected by the level of image noise inherent in a section of tissue.

The uniformity of CT numbers may vary temporally as well as spatially and should be monitored as part of a quality control program to evaluate the CT unit on a day-by-day basis. The reproducibility of CT numbers from one time to the next is especially important in repeated examinations of the same patient and in situations in which quantitative interpretations of CT numbers are attempted. In some CT units, it is necessary to determine the mean CT number for a water or plastic phantom and then scale all CT numbers obtained for patients either up or down, depending on the mean CT value for that particular day.

IMAGE NOISE

The term *image noise* refers to the random variation of CT numbers about some mean value when an image is obtained of a uniform object. This characteristic of a CT image imparts a graininess to the image that is particularly troublesome during visualization of low-contrast objects. Image noise can be described by the Wiener noise power spectrum, in which the noise is displayed as a function of spatial frequency [8, 15]; however, simpler methods such as computation of the standard deviation of the CT numbers usually are employed to describe image noise. This method is particularly simple and should be incorporated into a quality control program for the CT unit.

The principal source of noise in a CT image is *quantum mottle*, defined as the spatial and temporal statistical variation in the number of x rays absorbed in the detectors. Other sources of noise include round-off errors in the reconstruction program, electronic noise, and noise contributed by the display system. The pixel size of the display unit also influences image noise: larger pixels yield some reduction in image noise, possibly at the expense of spatial resolution. Many CT units offer *smoothing routines* in the reconstruction software to suppress the appearance of noise in the image. This suppression is accompanied by some degradation in spatial resolution.

Brooks and DiChiro [4] have described a relationship between image noise and the factors that influence this feature of CT images. The relationship is

$$\sigma^2 = \frac{K}{w^3 hD}$$

where σ is the standard deviation of the CT numbers constituting the image, w is the size of the individual volume elements (*voxels*), h is the thickness of the tissue section imaged by the CT unit, D is the amount of radiation used to produce the image, and K is a constant. From this relationship, several generalizations can be drawn: (1) image noise increases dramatically with decreasing size of the voxels used in the CT scanning process; (2) image noise increases with decreasing thickness of the tissue sections; and (3) image noise varies inversely with the amount of radiation used for the CT examination.

IMAGE DISTORTION AND ARTIFACTS

CT images are subject to artifacts and distortion arising from a variety of causes. Included among this category of image problems are such charac-

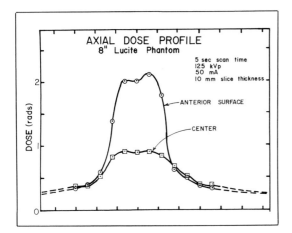

FIGURE 8-7. *Absorbed dose profiles at the surface and at midline of a patient examined with a fourth-generation CT unit.*

teristics as beam hardening and partial-volume artifacts that accompany all CT units. Also included are various streaklike artifacts produced by patient motion during an examination, by the presence of high-density objects in the patient, and by imbalanced detectors (in fourth-generation CT units). In third-generation scanners, imbalanced detectors create concentric-ring, rather than streak, artifacts; however, these are no less disturbing to the viewer. Display devices used with CT units often distort the image spatially, thereby introducing inaccuracies in spatial measurements obtained from the displayed image.

The evaluation of CT artifacts and distortion in a reliable and reproducible manner is a difficult problem that has not been entirely solved. The assessment of beam-hardening artifacts has been addressed by Duerinckx and Macovski [7] and by Joseph and Spital [11], and motion artifacts have been studied by Alfidi and co-workers [1]. Ibbott [10] has examined the problem of spatial distortion in CT viewing devices. The evaluation and elimination of artifacts and distortion in CT images are fruitful areas for further study.

ABSORBED DOSE IN COMPUTED TOMOGRAPHY

The radiation dose delivered to a patient during a CT examination varies from unit to unit and also over the section of tissue exposed during the examination. The variation of dose over the tissue section is especially notable for CT units with rotation limited to 180 degrees. Most measurements of absorbed dose are obtained with thermoluminescent dosimeters, although a multisegmented ionization chamber designed specifically for absorbed-dose measurements with CT units was recently introduced [14]. The absorbed dose delivered by a CT unit can be described by *dose profiles* obtained at various depths in a phantom. Shown in Figure 8-7 are

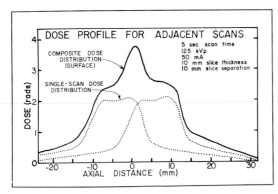

FIGURE 8-8. *Surface-absorbed dose profiles for sections of tissue adjacent to one another and examined with a fourth-generation CT unit. The dotted curve is the dose profile for examination of a single section.*

dose profiles at the surface and at midline for single section examination of a patient. These profiles were measured for a fourth-generation CT unit with 360-degree rotation of the x-ray tube. When adjacent tissue sections are irradiated, the dose profiles will increase somewhat because of radiation scattered into the section from adjacent tissues. The increase in dose when multiple adjacent sections of tissue are examined is illustrated in Figure 8-8. The absorbed dose delivered during a CT procedure depends primarily on the level of noise that can be tolerated in the image and on the efficiency with which the transmitted photons are utilized by the detectors (i.e., the *capture ratio*). Other factors include the kilovolt peak employed for the examination, the amount of overscan, if any, required to accelerate and decelerate the x-ray tube, the amount of off-focus radiation that is not utilized by the detectors, and the amount of filtration in the x-ray beam. Each of these factors should be examined for a CT unit, to ensure that adequate diagnostic information is being obtained with the lowest possible dose of radiation to the patient.

REFERENCES

1. Alfidi, R. H., MacIntyre, W. J., and Haaga, J. R. The effects of biological motion on CT resolution. *AJR* 127:11, 1976.
2. Bergstrom, M. Performance Evaluation of Scanners. In T. H. Newton and D. G. Potts (eds.), *Radiology of the Skull and Brain: Technical Aspects of Computed Tomography.* St. Louis: Mosby, 1981. P. 4212.
3. Brooks, R. A., and Di Chiro, G. Beam hardening in x-ray reconstructive tomography. *Phys. Med. Biol.* 21:390, 1976.
4. Brooks, R. A., and Di Chiro, G. Statistical limitations in x-ray reconstructive tomography. *Med. Phys.* 3:237, 1976.
5. Cohen, G., and DiBianca, F. A. The use of contrast-detail-dose evaluation of image quality in a computed tomographic scanner. *J. Comput. Assist. Tomogr.* 3:189, 1979.

6. Di Chiro, G., et al. The apical artifact: Elevated attenuation values toward the apex of the skull. *J. Comput. Assist. Tomogr.* 2:65, 1978.

7. Duerinckx, A. J., and Macovski, A. Polychromatic streak artifacts in computed tomography images. *J. Comput. Assist. Tomogr.* 2:481, 1978.

8. Hanson, K. M., and Boyd, D. P. The characteristics of computed tomographic reconstruction noise and their effect on detectability. *IEEE Trans. Nucl. Sci.* NS-25:160, 1978.

9. Hasegawa, B. H., et al. Problems with contrast-detail curves for CT performance evaluation. *AJR* 138:135, 1982.

10. Ibbott, G. S. Radiation therapy treatment planning and the distortion of CT images (letter to the editor). *Med. Phys.* 7:261, 1980.

11. Joseph, P. M., and Spital, R. D. A method for correcting bone-induced artifacts in computed tomography scanners. *J. Comput. Assist. Tomogr.* 2:100, 1978.

12. McCullough, E. C., et al. An evaluation of the quantitative and radiation features of a scanning x-ray transverse axial tomograph: The EMI scanner. *Radiology* 111:709, 1974.

13. McCullough, E. C. Photon attenuation in computed tomography. *Med. Phys.* 2:307, 1975.

14. Moore, M. M., Cacak, R. K., and Hendee, W. R. Multisegmented ion chamber for CT scanner dosimetry. *Med. Phys.* 8:640, 1981.

15. Riederer, S. J., Pelc, N. J., and Chesler, D. A. The noise power spectrum in computed x-ray tomography. *Phys. Med. Biol.* 23:446, 1978.

16. Rutherford, R. A., Pullan, B. R., and Isherwood, I. Calibration and response of an EMI scanner. *Neuroradiology* 11:7, 1976.

9

Image Clarity in Computed Tomography

In describing the clarity of information present in a radiologic image, one must consider four factors: spatial resolution, contrast resolution, image noise, and the presence of image distortion and artifacts [3]. Three of these factors and their influence on the computed tomographic (CT) image are considered in this chapter. The remaining influence, image distortion and artifacts, is discussed in the next chapter.

SPATIAL RESOLUTION

The ability of an imaging system to *resolve* (i.e., to portray as distinct entities) two small structures that are close together in the object is called the *spatial resolution* (or *resolving power*) of the system. Spatial resolution varies from one type of radiologic imaging system to another. For example, a chest x-ray unit employing a 1-mm focal spot, 180-cm target-film distance, and a detail-intensifying screen yields a spatial resolution of 0.1 to 0.2 mm. At the other extreme, clinical nuclear medicine images obtained with a modern scintillation camera provide a spatial resolution of 5 to 10 mm. The spatial resolution of CT images is intermediate between these extremes and usually is stated as 1 to 2 mm; modest improvements in these values are quoted for images from the newest CT units. This value of spatial resolution describes the lateral (i.e., the x-y) dimensions of the CT image; the third dimension of the image (i.e., the in-depth, or z, dimension) is determined by the thickness of the tissue section used to form the CT image.

The spatial resolution of a CT image is determined primarily by the collimation of the x-ray beam as it impinges on the radiation detectors. Other geometric influences on spatial resolution include the size of the focal spot of the x-ray tube and the axial position of the object between the x-ray tube and the detectors. Another, but usually less important, influence is the quality of the computer program used to reconstruct the image from measurements of x-ray transmission. In early CT units, relatively large detectors with rather coarse collimators were used in conjunction with pencil-like x-ray beams in either a parallel-beam or fan-beam configuration. As the geometry of the x-ray beam and the quality of the reconstruction programs improved during the early years of CT evolution, the collimator aperture in front of each radiation detector became the determining factor in spatial resolution. Consequently, smaller detectors were developed to interface with smaller collimators, with more detector-collimator pairs packed into the detector ring. Some of the more recent CT units contain more than 2,000 detector-collimator pairs positioned around a 360-degree ring, with each collimator transmitting an x-ray beam no larger than 1 mm in diameter onto the appropriate detector.

As smaller collimators and detectors are added to the detector ring, increased space is occupied by the collimators, and more x rays are absorbed in the collimating material. This absorption reduces the number of x rays available to form an image and leads to an increase in image noise. The increase in noise can be circumvented only by increasing the number of x rays used for a CT examination. This procedure increases both the patient dose and the heat generated in the x-ray tube (i.e., the *tube loading*). Achievement of an optimum balance among spatial resolution, image noise, patient dose, and tube loading is a challenge for manufacturers of CT units. This challenge has stimulated research on the design of new x-ray tubes with greater heat capacity, and the use of semiconductor radiation detectors with improved signal-to-noise ratios (the *signal-to-noise ratio* is the amplitude of the signal of interest divided by the amplitude of background noise).

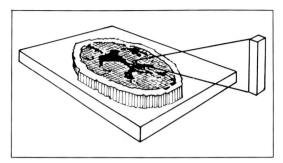

FIGURE 9-1.   *Each picture element (pixel) in the CT image corresponds to a volume element (voxel) of tissue in the patient. (Reprinted from E. C. McCullough, Factors affecting the use of quantitative information from a CT scanner. Radiology 124:99, 1977. With permission.)*

Distinction between the spatial resolution of a CT unit and that of the display device used with the unit often is a source of confusion. The spatial resolution (or resolving power) of a CT unit is a measured quantity (see Chapter 8) usually having a value of 1 to 2 mm. This value is affected severely by the reconstruction algorithm or display device only if too few attenuation values are computed by the algorithm or if the resolution of the display device is insufficient to display each of the computed values. Neither of these conditions is normally present in modern CT units.

A *display device* for CT can be described as a matrix of picture elements (*pixels*), with each pixel corresponding to a volume element (*voxel*) of tissue for which a CT number is computed. The relationship between pixels and voxels is depicted in Figure 9-1. The size of each pixel defines the resolution of the display device and can be estimated as shown in the following example.

Example. Suppose a 400-mm × 400-mm section of tissue is imaged on a display device composed of 512 × 512 pixels. Each pixel displays 400 mm/512 pixels or a 0.78-mm × 0.78-mm area of tissue. Hence, the spatial resolution of the display device is about 0.8 mm. This resolution is considerably better than the 1 to 2 mm value of spatial resolution characteristic of the image as influenced primarily by the detector collimators. It certainly would be inappropriate to describe the spatial resolution of the CT unit as 0.8 mm.

The third dimension of the CT image also is important in describing the clarity of information in the image. This dimension is the section thickness; it varies from 2 to 15 mm or so, usually at the discretion of the user. The section thickness is changed by varying the width of the x-ray beam: thinner sections are provided by a narrower x-ray beam. As the x-ray beam is narrowed, fewer x rays are used to form the image, and image noise is increased. This increase in noise can be circumvented only if the heat-loading characteristics of the x-ray tube permit more intense production of x rays.

As the section thickness is increased, greater thicknesses of tissue are presented as a two-dimensional image on the display device. For each volume element in the section, the CT number computed for the display pixel represents an average value for all tissue constituents in the voxel. For a voxel containing both muscle and bone, for example, the CT number is intermediate between values for muscle and bone weighted by the relative proportions of muscle and bone in the voxel. On the display device, this value will be presented as a shade of gray intermediate between those for bone and muscle. The resulting contrast distortion of the gray-scale image is known as the *partial-volume artifact;* it can be reduced only by using thinner sections to form the image. As was noted earlier, however, the use of thinner sections leads to an increase in image noise, because fewer photons are used to form the image.

CONTRAST RESOLUTION

Contrast resolution (or *low-contrast perceptibility*) refers to the ability of an imaging system to reveal slight differences in atomic composition or physical density in the patient. Compared to most other imaging modalities, CT provides superior contrast resolution. The contrast resolution of CT typically is 0.5 to 1 percent, signifying that differences of 0.5 to 1 percent in x-ray transmission through the patient are distinguishable in the image. This level of contrast resolution is superior to that in roentgenography, in which differences in x-ray transmission on the order of 5 percent are required before structures can be distinguished in the image.

The contrast resolution of CT images is superior to that in conventional roentgenography principally for three reasons. First, the image of a section of tissue is portrayed with no overlying or underlying structure; this characteristic is in contrast to conventional roentgenography, in which the entire thickness of the patient is superimposed on a two-dimensional image. Second, the use of solid-state detectors and ionization chambers in place of x-ray film provides a radiation detection system that is more sensitive to subtle changes in x-ray transmission. Third, there is little scatter radiation present in the highly collimated x-ray beam used in CT. All these factors combine to provide a level of contrast resolution in CT that far exceeds that in roentgenography and other imaging modalities.

In CT, contrast resolution is influenced primarily by the noise present in the CT image. The level of image noise is a reflection principally of the number of photons absorbed by the radiation detectors and used to form the final image. This limitation is known as quantum mottle and is influenced by a number of technique variables associated with image formation. Each of these influences is described in the next section.

IMAGE NOISE

Limitations in image reproducibility introduced by imprecision in the number of x rays used to form the image are referred to as *quantum mottle*. This imprecision is especially important in computed tomography, in which the contribution of quantum mottle to image noise is one of the major limitations in contrast resolution [1, 4, 5, 6, 7]. Quantum mottle is illustrated, somewhat simplistically, in the following example.

Example. A structure provides a 2 percent difference in x-ray transmission compared to the surrounding medium. In conventional roentgenography, how many x rays should be used to form an image such that the structure will be distinct from the surrounding medium with 95 percent confidence?

A 95 percent confidence level means that the structure will be distinctly different in 95 percent of all images. This confidence level corresponds to a 200

σ/N confidence interval, where σ/N represents the standard error in the number of x rays transmitted through the structure and absorbed in the detectors. The *standard error* is the estimated standard deviation σ of the number of x rays transmitted by the structure and absorbed in the detectors, divided by the number N of absorbed x rays. Since 200 $\sigma/N = 2$ percent, 100 $\sigma/N = 1$ percent or a fractional value of 0.01. The statistics of x-ray transmission follow a Poisson distribution law, where $\sigma = \sqrt{N}$. Therefore

$$\frac{\sqrt{N}}{N} = \frac{1}{\sqrt{N}} = 0.01$$

$$\sqrt{N} = \frac{1}{0.01} = 100$$

and

$$N = 10,000.$$

Therefore, 10,000 x rays must be transmitted by the structure and absorbed in the detectors if a 2 percent difference in transmission between the structure and the surrounding medium is to be revealed with 95 percent confidence. By the same reasoning, 100 x rays absorbed in the detectors would produce a much noisier image, and a 20 percent difference in transmission would be required before the structure could be distinguished from the surrounding medium with 95 percent confidence. Similarly, a transmission of 10^6 x rays would reveal a difference of 0.2 percent in x-ray transmission between the structure and the surrounding medium at a confidence level of 95 percent.

Although the above example illustrates the influence of quantum mottle in conventional roentgenographic imaging, it is too simplistic for CT images, primarily because structures are viewed from many orientations in CT. Also, a number of factors other than quantum mottle affect the noise level of CT images. Included among these factors are noise contributed by the radiation detectors (electronic noise) and by the reconstruction algorithm. The latter source of noise is due in part to round-off errors arising from the manipulation of numbers during the reconstruction process. Conceptually similar round-off errors occur during the display of gray-scale images in CT [2].

In CT, electronic noise and the noise contributed by the reconstruction process usually are less significant than quantum mottle. If these influences are relatively small, then the level of quantum mottle (i.e., noise) in the CT image should vary as $\sqrt{1/D}$, where D is the radiation dose to the patient.

REFERENCES

1. Hanson, K. M. Detectability in computed tomographic images. *Med. Phys.* 6:441, 1979.
2. Hanson, K. M. Noise and Contrast Discrimination in Computed Tomography. In T. H. Newton and D. G. Potts (eds.), *Radiology of the Skull and Brain: Technical Aspects of Computed Tomography*. St. Louis: Mosby, 1981. P. 3941.
3. Hendee, W. R., and Kuni, C. C. Concepts of Radiologic Imaging. Chicago: Year Book. In preparation.
4. Huesman, R. H. The effects of a finite number of projection angles and finite lateral sampling of projections on the propagation of statistical errors in transverse section reconstruction. *Phys. Med. Biol.* 22:511, 1977.
5. Joseph, P. M. Image noise and smoothing in computed tomography (CT) scanners. *Opt. Engr.* 17:396, 1978.
6. Riederer, S. J., Pelc, N. J., and Chesler, D. A. The noise power spectrum in computed x-ray tomography. *Phys. Med. Biol.* 23:446, 1978.

10

Artifacts in Computed Tomographic Images

Computed tomographic (CT) images frequently contain artifacts that reflect limitations in the image-forming process rather than disease within the patient. Artifacts may arise from various sources, including the x-ray tube, x-ray beam, patient, detectors, processing of transmission data, computation of CT values, display of these values as a gray-scale image, and manipulation of the contrast and density of the image. Some of these sources of artifacts and the characteristic patterns they produce in the image are discussed in this chapter.

SOFTWARE ARTIFACTS

Software artifacts are best explained by consideration of a first-generation CT scannner in which a *projection* (i.e., a set of x-ray transmission measurements at a single angle) can be easily distinguished from a *view* (i.e., any one of several angles at which transmission measurements are obtained). Although similar software artifacts occur with CT scanners of later vintage, fan-shaped x-ray beams and detectors moving in circular paths around the patient make the discussion of software artifacts more difficult.

Aliasing

The highest spatial frequency (i.e., the greatest number of lines per millimeter) that can be reproduced in a CT image defines the separation required between successive transmission measurements in a single projection for the image. This relationship is known as the *Nyquist criterion* and is stated as

$$d = \frac{1}{2\nu_0}$$

where d is the maximum desirable separation and ν_0 is the maximum spatial frequency. In general, ν_0 may be estimated as $1/(\text{FWHM})$, where FWHM is the full width at half max-

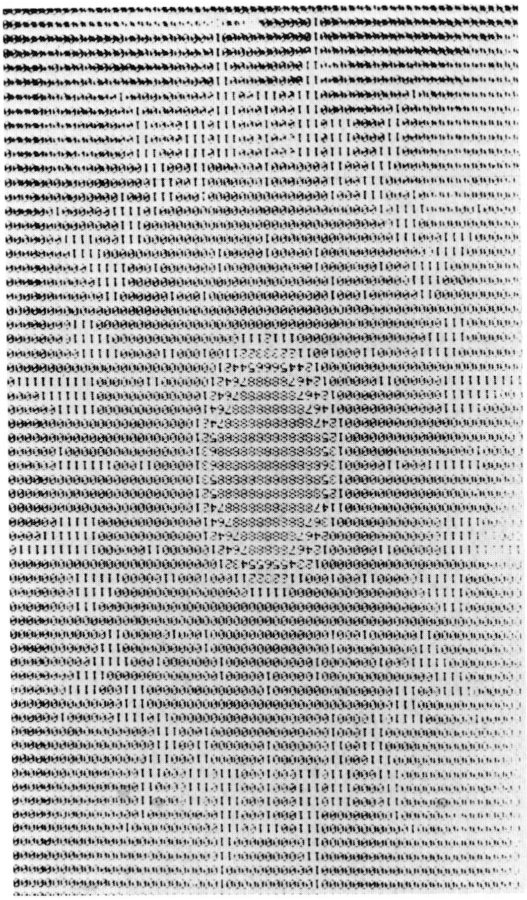

FIGURE 10-1. *Aliasing in a CT image caused by inadequate sampling of the object. (From G. A. Thieme, et al., Cross-sectional anatomic images by gamma-ray transmission scanning.* Acta Radiol. Oncol. Radiat. Phys. Biol. *14:81, 1975. With permission.)*

imum of the x-ray beam. For the pencil-like x-ray beam of a first-generation CT scanner, the FWHM is the width of the beam when the beam edges are defined by locations where the x-ray intensity is half that at beam center. In a single projection, the maximum separation between adjacent transmission measurements should not exceed half the FWHM for the x-ray beam. The total number n of transmission measurements is

$$n = D/d = 2D/(FWHM)$$

where D is the length of the projection (i.e., the lateral distance over which x-ray transmission measurements are obtained for a single projection). If transmission measurements are obtained at separations greater than the Nyquist criterion, high-frequency information is displaced, and the quality of the CT image is degraded. Furthermore, the displaced higher frequencies spuriously reappear at lower frequencies, creating an artifactual pattern referred to as aliasing. The term *aliasing* is used because the higher-frequency information appears "under an alias," as artifactual information at lower frequencies. In many CT images, aliasing artifacts may be small but still noticeable as tangential streaks near sharp boundaries in the images.

If the Nyquist criterion cannot be satisfied in a particular CT unit, the preferred solution is to lower the bandwidth (i.e., reduce the transmitted spatial frequencies by increasing the x-ray beam width) rather than to tolerate noticeable aliasing in the image. An example of aliasing is shown in Figure 10-1.

The number of views, or angular orientations, at which transmission data should be collected can also be predicted. The minimum number of views m is $m = n \pi/2$, where n is the number of transmission measurements per projection. The views should be equally spaced from 0 to at least 180°. If this sampling crite-

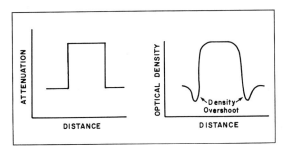

FIGURE 10-2.   *Illustration of the "reverse density" effect of the Gibbs phenomenon.*

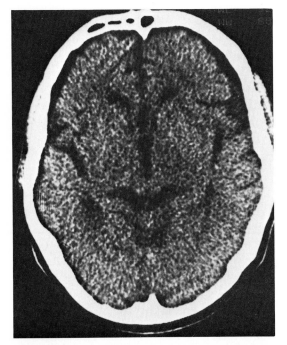

FIGURE 10-3.   *Head CT image displaying the Gibbs phenomenon as an artifactual ring of reduced physical density along the inner surface of the skull.*

rion is not satisfied, the image again may exhibit streak artifacts in the vicinity of sharp edges, especially near the periphery of the image. Sampling criteria for the number of views required for more complex scanner geometries are described in the literature [6, 11].

If more transmission measurements or views are obtained than are required by the criteria described above, the image is said to be *overdetermined*. For the overdetermined case, the image is reconstructed by averaging the redundant data, and noise in the image is reduced. All modern CT scanners furnish overdetermined images.

Gibbs Phenomenon

When spatial frequencies above a certain level (as defined, for example, by the x-ray beam width) are not reproduced in the CT image, another artifact may appear at sharp boundaries in the image. This artifact is called the *Gibbs phenomenon, algorithm overshoot, or ringing*. The Gibbs phenomenon is depicted in Figure 10-2, in which a sharp boundary in the object is depicted in the image as a gradient of optical density, with a density "overshoot" just inside the boundary. In Figure 10-3 this overshoot in optical density appears as a ring of reduced physical density (g/cm^3) just inside the skull. Artifacts caused by the Gibbs phenomenon were common in images produced by early CT scanners.

The Gibbs phenomenon can be suppressed by filtering the spatial frequencies so that a gradual "roll-off" of higher spatial frequencies occurs in place of a sharp cutoff. This filtering operation reduces the visibility of noise in the image, as well as the presence of the Gibbs phenomenon; however, it also degrades the spatial resolution of the image. The principle of applying a frequency roll-off filter is shown in Figure 10-4. Different types of frequency filters may be selected, depending on the trade-offs desired from among the competing factors of algorithm overshoot, noise, and spatial resolution [3, 9, 12]. On occasion, a certain amount of Gibbs phe-

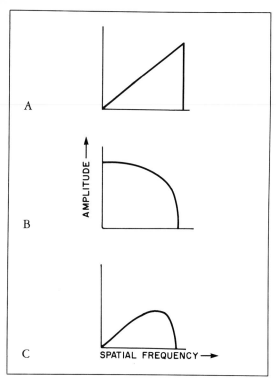

FIGURE 10-4. *A. A ramp or butterfly filter designed to transmit spatial frequencies up to a predetermined cutoff value. This filter provides reconstruction images subject to the Gibbs phenomenon. B. A smoothing filter designed to roll off higher spatial frequencies for suppression of noise and the Gibbs phenomenon. C. The product of A and B provides a modified ramp filter.*

nomenon may be desirable as a means of edge enhancement in the image.

BEAM GEOMETRY ARTIFACTS

Various image artifacts are associated with the geometry of the x-ray beam. Among the properties of the x-ray beam that contribute to image artifacts are the width and height of the x-ray beam, the nonuniformity of x-ray intensity across the x-ray beam, and the misalignment of the x-ray beam with respect to the radiation detectors. These problems have been discussed at length by R. A. Brooks and G. Di Chiro [1].

X-Ray Beam Width

In CT, the spatial resolution in the plane of the image (i.e., the lateral spatial resolution) is determined by the width of the x-ray beam admitted to each detector. Since this width is determined by the detector collimator, the aperture of the detector collimator determines the lateral spatial resolution in the CT image. A lesser influence on lateral resolution is the motion of the x-ray source and detectors during an x-ray attenuation measurement.

X-Ray Beam Height (Section Thickness)

The depth, or z-axis, resolution of a CT image is determined by the thickness of the section of tissue presented in the image. This thickness reflects the height of the x-ray beam exposing the section. Section thicknesses of about 1 cm are common in CT, so the depth resolution is typically poorer by a factor of 5 to 10 than the 1- to 2-mm lateral resolution present in most images. Although thinner sections can be obtained, they result in a reduction in the number of x rays used to form the image. Consequently, thin section images are inherently noisier than images of thicker sections.

Partial-Volume Artifact

A problem aggravated by the use of thick sections is the partial-volume artifact. Consider a voxel in a cross-sectional slice through the body. This voxel may contain tissues of various compositions, and the transmission of x rays through the voxel represents a weighted average of the transmission for each constituent of the voxel. Consequently, the linear attenuation coefficient μ computed for the voxel has an intermediate value

$$\mu = \frac{\mu_1 V_1 + \mu_2 V_2 + \ldots + \mu_n V_n}{V}$$

where $\mu_1, \mu_2, \ldots \mu_n$ are the linear attenuation coefficients for each of n tissue constituents occupying the voxel; $V_1, V_2 \ldots V_n$ are the volumes of each of the constituents in the voxel; and V is the total volume of the voxel. The attenuation coefficient μ and therefore its corresponding CT number have some intermediate value among those appropriate for each tissue constituent. This effect is known as the *partial-volume artifact*. The partial-volume artifact is particularly troublesome when quantitative interpretations of CT values are attempted in regions where tissue densities are changing rapidly and where, to suppress noise, relatively thick sections are required.

X-Ray Intensity Variations

Another problem attributable to the x-ray beam is caused by spatial and temporal variations in x-ray intensity in the beam. These variations are a reflection of the random nature of x-ray production and interaction and the divergent nature of the x-ray beam; they depend in part on the geometry of the x-ray source and the source and detector collimators. Nonuniform x-ray intensities are accentuated in scanner geometries that employ adjacent detectors to obtain data simultaneously for two contiguous sections of tissue. The effect of variations in x-ray intensity caused by a divergent x-ray beam is depicted in Figure 10-5.

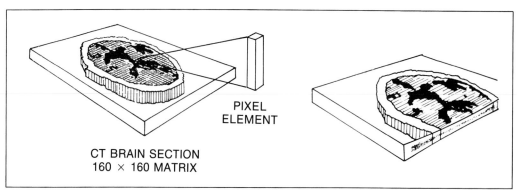

PIXEL
ELEMENT

CT BRAIN SECTION
160 × 160 MATRIX

FIGURE 10-5. *Two conceptions of the tomographic "slice."* Left: *Idealized slice with uniform thickness and sensitivity. (Courtesy of Dr. Thomas Payne, University of Minnesota.)* Right: *Realistic slice, shown cut in half so that variation in thickness may be better seen. In this example, slice is thinner in the center. The shading along the cut edge indicates that the sensitivity is greatest along the midplane and least at the upper and lower surfaces. (From R. A. Brooks, and G. Di Chiro, Slice geometry in computer assisted tomography.* J. Comput. Assist. Tomogr. *1:191, 1977. With permission.)*

X-Ray Beam Misalignment

Misalignment of the x-ray beam with respect to the radiation detectors creates a pattern of streaks at the boundaries of high-density structures in the image. This pattern resembles the streak artifacts resulting from gradual motion of the patient and can be distinguished only by a test procedure utilizing high-density pins in a stationary object [5]. In third- and fourth-generation CT units, software routines usually are used to correct for misalignment of the multiple radiation detectors with respect to the target of the x-ray tube. A different artifactual pattern known as the *"tuning fork" artifact* is caused by misalignment of the rotational center of the x-ray beam with respect to the axis of the coordinate system used for reconstruction [10].

BEAM HARDENING

If transmission measurements for CT were obtained with a monoenergetic beam of photons, all locations in the object would be sampled with photons of the same energy and all attenuation coefficients would be appropriate for that particular energy. To reduce image noise, however, large numbers of photons are needed in CT, and sources of monoenergetic radiation such as radionuclides are not practical. Instead, polyenergetic x-ray beams from conventional x-ray tubes are used to obtain transmission measurements in CT. In the image, these sources produce an artifactual pattern known as *beam hardening*.

As a narrow polyenergetic x-ray beam traverses an object in CT, lower-energy x rays interact more frequently and are selectively removed from the x-ray beam. Consequently, the average energy of the x-ray beam increases with depth in the object, and the corresponding attenuation coefficients decrease in value. This process is referred to as beam hardening; it results in a nonuniform pattern of attenuation coefficients across the object, which produces

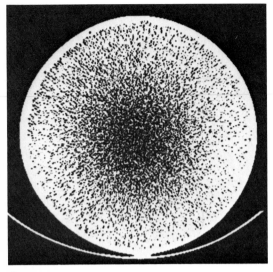

A

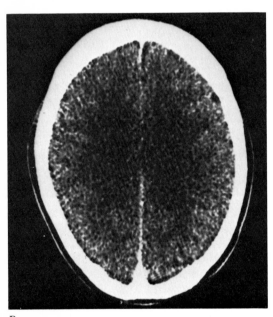

B

FIGURE 10-6. *Beam hardening. A. Image of a uniform phantom. B. Image of a patient.*

different CT numbers in different regions of an object of uniform composition.

By scanning an object from many different directions, the beam hardening artifact can be reduced but not eliminated. The "cupping" artifact, in which CT numbers at the center of an image are lower than those at the periphery of a uniform object scanned from all directions (i.e., 360 degrees), is a reflection of beam hardening [2, 13]. For symmetrical geometries such as a ring of bone surrounding homogeneous soft tissue (e.g., the skull), approximate corrections for beam hardening can be applied as the transmission data are processed for image reconstruction [4, 7, 8]. For less symmetrical, more inhomogeneous objects, beam-hardening corrections applied during the postprocessing stage of image reconstruction are less satisfactory. The beam-hardening artifact is illustrated in Figure 10-6.

Another contribution to beam hardening is the variable path-length of the x-ray beam through an asymmetrical object as the object is scanned from different directions. To provide an x-ray path of constant length for all orientations of the x-ray beam, some early CT scanners employed a water bag secured tightly around the scanned region. More recent CT scanners have eliminated the water bag because it is bulky and inconvenient for the patient. To reduce beam hardening caused by variable lengths of the x-ray path through the patient, these scanners employ various filters and software routines.

DETECTOR AND MOTION ARTIFACTS

Among the common artifacts in CT images are the streaks and swirls contributed by imbalanced detectors. Reduction of these artifacts is the principal reason for the elaborate care taken before and during an examination to ensure that all the detectors exhibit nearly the same sensitivity to impinging radiation. Typical patterns

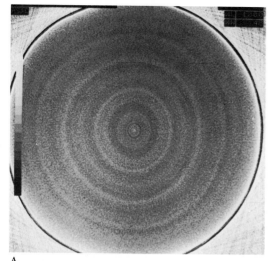

A

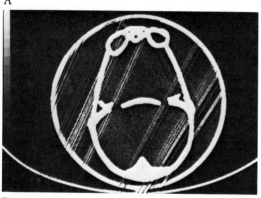

B

FIGURE 10-7.   *Artifacts caused by imbalanced detectors. A. Spiral artifacts in a third-generation scanner. B. Streak artifacts in a fourth-generation scanner.*

caused by imbalanced detectors are shown in Figure 10-7.

Also encountered frequently in CT images are the streak artifacts characteristic of motion of the patient during the examination. These artifacts originate at the boundaries of bone or air- or gas-filled cavities and at the edges of other objects such as metal clips and pins that have physical densities greatly different from soft tissue. Motion artifacts can be reduced only by collecting the transmission data over a shorter interval of time. For this reason, motion artifacts are less frequent in images from the newer CT units with faster scan times.

REFERENCES

1. Brooks, R. A., and Di Chiro, G. Slice geometry in computer-assisted tomography. *J. Comput. Assist. Tomogr.* 1:191, 1977.
2. Brooks, R. A., and Di Chiro, G. Principles of computer-assisted tomography (CAT) in radiographic and radioisotopic imaging. *Phys. Med. Biol.* 21:689, 1976.
3. Chesler, D. A., and Riederer, S. J. Ripple suppression during reconstruction in transverse tomography. *Phys. Med. Biol.* 20:632, 1975.
4. Joseph, P. M., and Spital, R. D. A method for correcting bone-induced artifacts in computed tomography scanners. *J. Comput. Assist. Tomogr.* 2:100, 1978.
5. Joseph, P. M. Artifacts in Computed Tomography. In T. H. Newton and D. G. Potts (eds.), *Radiology of the Skull and Brain: Technical Aspects of Computed Tomography.* St. Louis: Mosby, 1981. P. 3956.
6. Logan, B. F. The uncertainty principle in reconstructing functions from projection. *Duke Math. J.* 42:661, 1975.
7. Nalcioglu, O., and Lou, R. Y. Postreconstruction method for beam hardening in computerized tomography. *Phys. Med. Biol.* 24:330, 1979.
8. Rüegsegger, P., et al. Standardization of computed tomography images by means of a material-selective beam-hardening correction. *J. Comput. Assist. Tomogr.* 1:184, 1978.

9. Sharp, J., Tiemann, J., and King, R. In *Image Processing for 2-D and 3-D Reconstruction from Projections*. Stanford: Opt. Soc. Am. 1975. P. THA 10-1.

10. Shepp, L. A., Hilal, S. K., and Schulz, R. A. The tuning fork artifact in reconstruction tomography. *Comput. Graphics Image Proc.* 10:246, 1979.

11. Snyder, D. L., and Cox, J. R., Jr. An Overview of Reconstructive Tomography and Limitations Imposed by a Finite Number of Projections. In M. M. Ter-Pogossian, et al. (eds.), *Reconstruction Tomography in Diagnostic Radiology and Nuclear Medicine*. Baltimore: University Press, 1977. P. 28.

12. Tanaka, E., and Iinuma, T. A. Correction functions for optimizing the reconstructed image in transverse section scan. *Phys. Med. Biol.* 20:789, 1975.

13. Zatz, L. M., and Alvarez, R. E. An inaccuracy in computed tomography: The energy dependence of CT values. *Radiology* 124:91, 1977.

11 Quantitative Interpretation of Computed Tomography Data

As was stated in Chapter 2, computed tomography (CT) numbers are related directly to the linear attenuation coefficients appropriate for the effective energy (keV) of the x-ray beam used to obtain the CT numbers. Since linear attenuation coefficients for soft tissues are a direct reflection of volume electron densities (electrons/cm^3) and, more fundamentally, of mass densities (g/cm^3) within an accuracy of 2 percent or so, the potential exists to characterize soft tissues by analysis of their CT numbers. To date, this potential has been realized only superficially in clinical applications of CT, primarily because of statistical uncertainties and physical artifacts present in CT data. These limitations are discussed in this chapter, together with the prospects for their resolution so that quantitative CT may become a reality. The discussion is approached by presenting CT measurements on excised tissues where the presence of physical artifacts can be minimized. This section is followed by discussion of the difficulties associated with in vivo compilation of quantitative CT data, in which physical artifacts are less controllable. The final section covers some of the statistical problems associated with the quantitative interpretation of CT data.

IN VITRO CT MEASUREMENTS

By making in vitro CT measurements on excised tissues, one can eliminate many of the physical artifacts associated with in vivo scanning. For example, beam-hardening artifacts can be minimized by positioning a small sample of tissue in a cylindrical water-filled phantom that is centered with respect to the geometry of the scanner. Motion and partial-volume artifacts can be eliminated by careful preparation of the sample, and other physical effects that reduce the reliability of CT measurements can be minimized by similar approaches. In some earlier CT scanners, these approaches were mimicked by surrounding the patient's anatomy with a water bag to minimize beam hardening and to restrict the detector signals to a range that the scanners could handle. Later scanners are more tolerant of beam hardening, can handle a wider range of detector signals, and have discarded the water bag.

In early in vitro measurements of CT data, difficulties were encountered in obtaining CT numbers that were near those predicted theoretically for different tissues. In most cases, the disagreements were caused by improper calibration of the CT scale. To obtain better agreement between measured and predicted CT values, R. A. Brooks [3] has suggested that the CT number for tissue samples be computed from the expression

$$\text{CT number} = 1{,}000 \, \frac{(CT)_T - (CT)_W}{(CT)_W - (CT)_A}$$

where the CT values within the brackets represent values measured for tissue (T), water (W), and air (A). With this approach, measured CT values can be normalized individually to a Hounsfield-unit (HU) scale, in which CT = 0 for water and CT = −1,000 for air.

In any in vitro measurement of tissue samples, a number of problems can arise that are related to the way the samples are handled. Among these problems are changes in the tissue samples caused by the differences in temperature between the samples in vivo and the samples at the time of the in vitro CT measurements; the presence of gas released during deterioration of the sample; the techniques employed for sample preservation; the loss of fluid from the sample; and the presence of a contrast medium in the samples. Although none of these problems is particularly new, their effects on CT values have been documented by a number of authors [4, 16, 19, 23] and should always be considered during in vitro measurements.

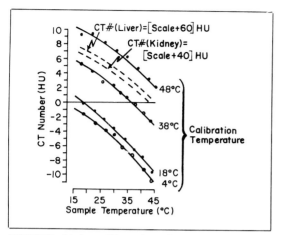

FIGURE 11-1. *CT numbers of water (solid curves) versus temperature for four temperatures of a calibration water phantom. Dotted lines show similar data for pig liver and kidney measured with a calibration temperature of 18°C. (Reprinted from G. D. Fullerton, Fundamentals of CT Tissue Characterization. In G. D. Fullerton and J. A. Zagzebski {eds.}, Medical Physics of CT and Ultrasound: Tissue Imaging and Characterization. New York: American Institute of Physics, 1980. P. 125. With permission.)*

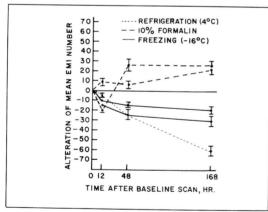

FIGURE 11-2. *Changes in CT number (EMI units) for tissues preserved by various methods and measured at three intervals over a week, with each number normalized to a baseline value of 0 for freshly excised, nonpreserved tissue. (Reprinted from J. Wittenberg, CT of in vitro abdominal organs—effects of preservation methods on attenuation coefficient. Comput. Tomogr. 1:95, 1977. With permission.)*

In early efforts to measure CT values for in vitro samples, problems were encountered because the temperature of the tissue samples was not carefully controlled. The effect of varying temperature of the sample, or of the water used to establish a reference value for the CT number scale, is shown in Figure 11-1, in which data have been replotted by G. D. Fullerton [8] from measurements obtained by G. M. Bydder and L. Kreel [4]. When the temperature is raised from 18 to 38°C, the CT value decreases by 6.5 HU for water, and by about 4.8 HU for pig liver and kidney. Hence, the temperature of tissue samples and water-calibration phantoms must be controlled carefully when in vitro measurements of tissue CT characteristics are attempted.

As soon as tissue is excised from a living organism, changes begin to occur that may affect the CT number for the tissue. For example, fluid, such as blood from an organ or urine from the kidneys, may be lost, causing a reduction in CT number in the first instance and an increase in CT number in the second. Often, the tissue is drained of fluid before in vitro CT measurements are attempted. Some of the possible effects of tissue preservation techniques on CT numbers are revealed in Figure 11-2, in which data are plotted in EMI units, with CT = −500 for air and 0 for water.

Because of the influence of various extraneous factors on CT numbers during the preparation of tissue samples, CT values obtained for particular categories of tissue specimens have shown poor agreement with each other and with CT values for the samples computed theoretically. This lack of agreement is due, at least in part, to different calibrations of the CT-number scale and to different methods of preparing the samples for measurement.

Another reason for variability in CT numbers is the difference in composition of similar tissues from different subjects. Shown in Figure 11-3 is the strong dependence of the mass density of adipose tissue on the water content of the tissue.

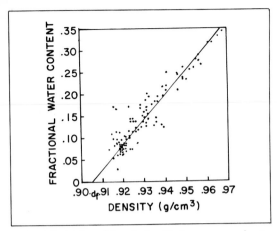

FIGURE 11-3. *The relationship between mass density (g/cm³) and water content for human fatty tissue. (Reprinted from T. H. Allen, H. J. Kryzwicki, and J. E. Roberts, Density, fat, water and solids in freshly isolated tissues. J. Appl. Physiol. 14:1005, 1959. With permission.)*

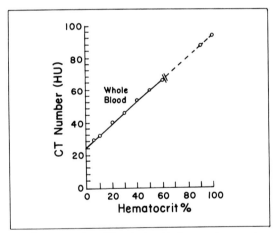

FIGURE 11-4. *The relationship between hematocrit and CT number for human blood (modified from P. F. J. New and S. Aronow, Attenuation measurements of whole blood and blood fractions in computed tomography. Radiology 121:635, 1976. With permission.)*

If the density values in Figure 11-3 are converted to corresponding CT numbers, variations as large as 50 HU are encountered in CT numbers for human adipose tissue. As another example, the CT number for blood varies significantly with the hematocrit for males above 14 years of age (Figure 11-4). The hematocrit for adult males often is assumed to be 47 percent, corresponding to a CT value of 58 HU. Actually, the hematocrit for males varies from 35 to 50 percent, corresponding to a CT-number range of 50 to 66 [15]. Women have a mean hematocrit of 42 percent, which corresponds to an average CT value of 54 HU. Since the hematocrit varies with altitude, the CT value for blood also varies with this factor.

IN VIVO CT MEASUREMENTS

When tissues for which CT information is desired remain in the body, the processes of sample handling and measurement are greatly simplified. However, other problems arise that are equally, if not more, severe in the way they jeopardize the reliability of CT numbers. Among these problems are artifacts introduced by patient motion, beam hardening, and reconstruction errors, as well as errors caused by partial volume effects and pixel averaging. All these factors usually are present during in vivo studies, and they all contribute to errors in the CT value for a particular tissue.

Beam hardening is present in any CT image obtained with a polyenergetic x-ray beam. To compensate for beam hardening during quantitative CT measurements, most manufacturers recommend that scans be obtained for plastic or water-filled cylinders of various diameters corresponding to an adult head, adult torso, pediatric head, or other body part. From the relative values of CT numbers along the radial dimensions of these phantoms, beam-hardening corrections can be obtained, which normalize the CT numbers for patients of a given size. These corrections are not exact, and the CT values for a particular patient may be underestimated or overestimated by using beam-hardening corrections for a phantom of size similar to that of the patient. Moreover, the phantom is a homogeneous structure and does not exactly simulate the internal anatomy of the patient. All of these problems contribute to "cupping" and "capping" artifacts, in which the CT numbers for a particular tissue are lower or higher than they should be.

Various approaches have been taken to determine the overall reliability of CT numbers measured in vivo. In one approach, an anthropomorphic phantom was designed to simulate human soft tissues in the thorax [9]. Cross-sectional attenuation data for this phantom were obtained by scanning with six different CT scanners, and the CT numbers for the various tissues were compared to the ideal numbers computed from the known composition of the phantom. For the heart-stimulating material, the mean discrepancy was 9 ± 6 HU, with CT numbers ranging from 2 to 19 HU.

In another study, Bydder and Kreel [5] compared in vivo CT measurements of collections of abdominal fluids to in vitro CT analyses of the same fluids after they had been aspirated from the abdomen. The mean difference between the two measurements was 8 ± 6.5 HU, with a range of 0.2 to 22 HU. These results, as well as those from the anthropomorphic phantom study, illustrate the rather wide range of CT numbers that must be tolerated for a given tissue, at least with the equipment and techniques presently available for quantitative CT. This range may be subject to some reduction for certain anatomic regions where there is greater uniformity in tissues and in geometry from one patient to another. In a study of more than 60 apparently normal individuals, for example, Arimitsu [1] demonstrated a standard deviation of only 2.2 HU from the mean CT value for brain tissue. Because of the reduced variability

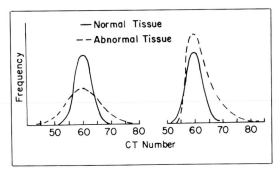

FIGURE 11-5. *Representation of the rationale for using statistics other than the mean CT number for identifying tissue pathology.* Left: *Change in range or standard deviation.* Right: *Change in skewness.* (*Modified from G. D. Fullerton, Fundamentals of CT Tissue Characterization. In G. D. Fullerton and J. A. Zagzebski {eds.},* Medical Physics of CT and Ultrasound: Tissue Imaging and Characterization. *New York: American Institute of Physics, 1980. P. 125. With permission.*)

in CT numbers for the brain as compared to most other anatomic regions, it is likely that this organ will be one of the first regions of patient anatomy to benefit significantly from quantitative CT [7, 13].

A few investigators have suggested that some indicator other than the mean CT number might be a more meaningful quantitative index of a tissue sample [12, 18]. Such an indicator might be the standard deviation, range, or skewness of the CT numbers associated with the tissue, as illustrated in Figure 11-5. To date, this approach has not yielded CT values that are sufficiently indicative of disease to be useful clinically.

A second approach to an indicator other than the mean CT value involves analysis of the degree of correlation of a particular CT value with its neighbors. In this fashion, the gradient of CT numbers can be examined, or an autocorrelation coefficient can be computed for a set of CT numbers [17, 20]. These approaches, however, have not been particularly successful clinically. The principal difficulties with alternative statistics are the variability in CT numbers for the same tissue from one CT unit to the next, and the wide range of numbers for normal tissues on the same unit.

CLINICAL APPLICATIONS OF QUANTITATIVE CT

Compared to the abdomen, the brain presents a more predictable pattern of CT numbers, and most applications of quantitative CT have been directed to this organ [12, 18]. Reproduced in Table 11-1 are CT numbers for white and gray matter of the brain taken from an article by Arimitsu and co-workers [1]. These data agree well with predicted CT numbers and with values reported by other investigators.

After a severe blow to the head, a hemorrhage may develop in which blood collects to form a hematoma. Shown in Figure 11-6 is the change in CT number as blood collects over the first 24

Table 11-1.   *Hounsfield Values for Various Regions in the Brain as Measured on the EMI CT1010**

Brain Region	Before Contrast (60 cases)	After Contrast (24 cases)	Contrast Enhancement (24 cases)
Gray matter			
Caudate nucleus	39.3 ± 2.3	41.7 ± 2.6	2.3 ± 1.9
Lenticular nucleus	38.9 ± 2.2	40.9 ± 2.6	1.8 ± 2.0
Thalamus	37.8 ± 2.0	39.4 ± 1.7	1.7 ± 1.5
Average	38.7 ± 2.2	40.7 ± 2.4	1.9 ± 1.8
White matter			
Subfrontal	33.0 ± 2.5	33.9 ± 2.7	1.1 ± 2.4
Centrum semiovale	32.5 ± 2.4	34.6 ± 3.0	1.8 ± 3.4
Forceps major	30.1 ± 2.0	31.3 ± 1.7	1.3 ± 2.0
Average	31.8 ± 2.3	33.2 ± 2.6	1.4 ± 2.3

*The ± values are standard deviations taken over the patient population. The contrast enhancement was measured for individual cases and then averaged over the patient population.

Source: Reprinted from T. Arimitsu, et al. White-gray matter differentiation in computed tomography. *J. Comput. Assist. Tomogr.* 1:437, 1977. With permission.

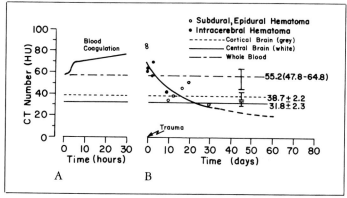

FIGURE 11-6.   *Variation of CT numbers during the formation and dissolution of a brain hematoma. A. In vitro measurements of CT number change during formation of a blood clot. B. In vivo decrease in CT number during dissolution of a brain hematoma. (Reprinted from G. D. Fullerton, Fundamentals of CT Tissue Characterization. In G. D. Fullerton and J. A. Zagzebski {eds.}, Medical Physics of CT and Ultrasound: Tissue Imaging and Characterization. New York: American Institute of Physics, 1980. P. 125. With permission.)*

hours and then is slowly reabsorbed. Normal human blood has a CT number of about 58, as shown on the left in Figure 11-6. As a hematoma develops, the blood clots into a mass consisting almost entirely of red blood cells, with a CT value near 90. In the region of the hematoma, the CT numbers return to values characteristic of white matter as the hematoma is absorbed slowly over days following its formation.

In a study by S. S. Siegelman and co-workers [22], CT numbers associated with pulmonary nodules in 88 patients were evaluated to identify quantitative criteria to distinguish benign from malignant lesions. For each nodule, a mean CT number was computed for the 32 volume elements with the highest CT number. For primary malignancies, the mean value was 92 ± 18 HU. The highest mean CT number was 147 HU for malignant lesions, whereas most of the benign lesions had a mean value of 164 HU or greater. Diffuse calcification probably was responsible for the higher mean CT number in benign lesions. The authors suggest that distinction of malignant from benign pulmonary lesions may be one clinical application of quantitative CT.

One approach to the use of CT to determine the chemical properties of tissues is the dual–kilovolt peak (kVp) technique. In this approach, x-ray transmission data measured at two different kVp settings are analyzed to yield the atomic number and electron density distributions within a region of interest in the patient. The dual-kVp technique for identification of the physical properties of biologic tissues is limited primarily by uncertainties in the small differences between CT numbers measured at the two settings. The dual-kVp technique has been used for studies in the brain [6, 14] and the liver [11], as well as for a variety of subtraction methods described in Chapter 13. Quantitative densitometry with single- and dual-kVp CT techniques also has been used for measurements of bone mineralization in the spines of normal patients, and for patients with suspected metabolic bone disease [2, 10]. Bone mineralization measurements also have been conducted with transmission-CT units employing a γ-emitting radioactive source in place of the x-ray tube [21]. These units provide a monoenergetic beam that is less susceptible to intensity fluctuations from moment to moment; however, the beam intensity is rather low, and examination times are long.

Another quantitative application of CT is determination of the linear dimension, area, and volume of anatomic structures under both static and dynamic conditions. In this application, the major difficulty is recognition of the exact boundary of the structure or structures of interest. This difficulty is currently the subject of intense scrutiny by a number of investigators, and improvements in boundary-recognition algorithms are expected in the near future.

Other applications of quantitative CT have been limited by the wide range in CT numbers for specific types of tissues, the variation in CT numbers for a particular tissue from one day (or hour) to the next, and the influence of artifacts such as pixel averaging, motion blurring, and beam hardening on this range of CT values. As corrections for these artifacts are improved, and as more baseline data are accumulated on normal tissue characteristics, additional applications of quantitative CT can be anticipated.

REFERENCES

1. Arimitsu, T., et al. White-gray matter differentiation in computed tomography. *J. Comput. Assist. Tomogr.* 1:437, 1977.
2. Boyd, D. B., et al. A proposed dynamic cardiac 3-D densitometer for early detection and evaluation of heart disease. *IEEE Trans. Nucl. Sci.* NS-26:2724, 1979.
3. Brooks, R. A. A quantitative theory of the Hounsfield unit and its application to dual-energy scanning. *J. Comput. Assist. Tomogr.* 1:487, 1977.

4. Bydder, G. M., and Kreel, L. The temperature dependence of computed tomography attenuation values. *J. Comput. Assist. Tomogr.* 3:506, 1979.

5. Bydder, G. M., and Kreel, L. Attenuation values of fluid collections within the abdomen. *J. Comput. Assist. Tomogr.* 4:145, 1980.

6. Di Chiro, G., et al. Tissue signatures with dual-energy computed tomography. *Radiology* 131:521, 1979.

7. Dubal, L., and Wiggli, U. Tomochemistry of the brain. *J. Comput. Assist. Tomogr.* 1:300, 1977.

8. Fullerton, G. D. Fundamentals of CT Tissue Characterization. In G. D. Fullerton and J. A. Zagzebski (eds.), *Medical Physics of CT and Ultrasound: Tissue Imaging and Characterization.* New York: American Institute of Physics, 1980. P. 125.

9. Fullerton, G. D., and White, D. R. Anthropomorphic test objects for CT scanners. *Radiology* 133:217, 1979.

10. Genant, H. K., et al. Quantitative Bone-Mineral Analysis Using Computed Tomography in Noninvasive Measurements of Bone Mass and Their Clinical Applications. In S. Cohn (ed.), *Noninvasive Measurements of Bone Mass and Their Clinical Applications.* New York: CRC Press, 1981.

11. Goldberg, H. I. Differential diagnosis of diffuse liver disease with use of dual-energy CT. *J. Comput. Assist. Tomogr.* 3:858, 1979.

12. Kramer, R. A., et al. Statistical profiles in computed tomography. *Radiology* 125:145, 1977.

13. Latchau, R. E., Payne, J. T., and Gold, L. H. A. Effective atomic number and electron density as measured with a computed tomographic scanner: Computation and correlation with brain tumor histology. *J. Comput. Assist. Tomogr.* 2:199, 1978.

14. Marshall, W. H., et al. Dual kilovoltage applied to CT: Determination of electron density effective atomic number and optimum reconstruction keV. *Proceedings of the 27th Annual Meeting of the AUR,* Rochester, N.Y., 1979.

15. New, P. F. J., and Aronow, S. Attenuation measurements of whole blood and blood fractions in computed tomography. *Radiology* 121:635, 1976.

16. Phelps, M. D., Hoffman, E. J., and Ter-Pogossian, M. M. Attenuation coefficients of various body tissues, fluid, and lesions at photon energies of 18 to 136 keV. *Radiology* 117:573, 1975.

17. Pullan, B. R., Fawcitt, R. A., and Isherwood, I. Tissue characterization by an analysis of the distribution of attenuation values in computed tomography scans. *J. Comput. Assist. Tomogr.* 2:49, 1978.

18. Reid, M. H., and Dublin, A. B. Statistical detection of nonvisible isodense subdural fluid collections. *J. Comput. Assist. Tomogr.* 3:491, 1979.

19. Rieth, K. G., et al. Serial measurements of CT attenuation and specific gravity in experimental cerebral edema. *Radiology* 135:343, 1980.

20. Ritchings, R. T., et al. An analysis of the spatial distribution of attenuation values in computed tomography scans of liver and spleen. *J. Comput. Assist. Tomogr.* 3:36, 1979.

21. Rüegsegger, P., et al. Quantification of bone mineralization using computed tomography. *Radiology* 121:93, 1976.

22. Siegelman, S. S., et al. CT of the solitary pulmonary nodule. *AJR* 135:1, 1980.

23. Wittenberg, J., et al. Computerized tomography of in vitro abdominal organs—effects of preservation methods on attenuation coefficient. *Comput. Tomogr.* 1:95, 1977.

12 Computed Tomography in Planning Radiotherapy Treatments

For a course of radiation therapy to be successful, the dose of radiation delivered to a tumor must be sufficient to destroy all the cells in the tumor. At the same time, normal tissues surrounding the tumor should receive much smaller amounts of radiation, so that few, if any, noncancerous cells are damaged by the radiation. These objectives require the careful planning of radiation treatments, and computed tomography (CT) is widely acknowledged as a major contributor to the planning effort. In almost all major centers for cancer treatment by radiation therapy, CT is recognized as an essential tool in the design and implementation of radiation treatments.

CT contributes to radiotherapy treatment planning in many ways. The location and extension of a tumor often can be delineated more accurately by CT than by any other imaging modality. Surrounding normal tissues also can be identified, and their attenuation coefficients can be determined so that the influence of these tissues on the distribution of radiation dose can be estimated. The external contour of the patient can be demarcated more accurately by CT than by any alternative technique currently available. The response of the tumor to irradiation can be monitored during the course of treatment to facilitate changes in the treatment plan whenever appropriate.

TUMOR LOCALIZATION

One of the major limitations in radiation therapy is the uncertainty in defining the exact margins of the tumor to be treated. Tumor recurrences often are attributed to inadequate irradiation of tissues that originally were thought to be free of cancerous cells. With CT, tumor boundaries often can be identified more exactly, so that a more satisfactory treatment plan can be designed to encompass all the affected tissue. The treatment plan can be designed in three dimensions with the help of coronal and sagittal CT images reconstructed from CT data accumulated in the transaxial plane.

Several investigators have evaluated the ability of computed tomography to improve the distribution of radiation dose in the region of a tumor. For example, J. E. Munzenrider and co-workers [24] concluded in a retrospective study that CT was essential to the treatment of 41 (55%) out of 76 patients. At the Royal Marsden Hospital in London, J. S. MacDonald and co-workers found that 21 out of 28 patients required a change in their treatment plan after evaluation by CT [19]. In a prospective study at Massachusetts General Hospital, M. Goitein and co-workers [11] reported that CT revealed inadequate treatment of tumors in 40 (52%) of 77 patients with treatment plans designed without CT. Improvements in treatment plans contributed by CT were reported for 64 percent of 45 patients examined by D. P. Ragan and C. A. Perez [29]. Of 72 patients scheduled for radiation therapy of pelvic cancer, CT techniques used by H. E. Brizel and co-workers [5] revealed that more than 40 percent had tumors larger than expected or had unsuspected invasions into normal tissue. In addition, these authors reported that tumor stages were revised upward in 25 percent of the patients. On the basis of follow-up studies of a number of patients with lung tumors, P. Van Houtte and colleagues [35] documented that CT improves treatment planning.

In spite of the accolades accorded to the use of CT in tumor identification and localization, there are also limitations in the application. For example, similarities in physical and electron densities between tumors and normal tissues often prevent the exact delineation of boundaries between the two types of tissues and the detection of invasions of tumor into normal tissue. This limitation is enhanced by partial-volume artifacts, and the poorer spatial resolution of coronal and sagittal CT images [20].

TISSUE CHARACTERIZATION

CT provides a two-dimensional matrix of CT numbers for a section of tissue through the patient. As discussed earlier, these CT numbers are related to linear attenuation coefficients μ by the relationship

$$CT \text{ number} = k \left(\frac{\mu - \mu_w}{\mu_w} \right)$$

where μ_w is the linear attenuation coefficient of water and k is a constant with a value of 1,000 for CT numbers expressed in Hounsfield units. From this relationship, the attenuation coefficient μ can be computed as

$$\mu = \mu_w \left(\frac{CT \text{ number} + k}{k} \right)$$

where μ is seen to vary directly with the CT number, provided that μ_w remains constant. R. A. Geise and E. C. McCullough [10] have demonstrated that for tissues other than bone, the ratio μ/μ_w varies essentially linearly with the volume electron density $(\rho_e)_v$ in units of electrons/cm^3. Therefore,

$$(\rho_e)_v = \frac{CT \text{ number} + k}{k}$$

and the cross-sectional distribution of CT numbers can be recomputed with reasonable accuracy ($\pm 3\%$) as a cross section of volume electron densities for soft tissue structures in the absence of bone. This conclusion has been verified by M. E. Phelps [27]; however, S. C. Prasad and co-workers [28] have shown that the relationship cannot be extended with similar accuracy to a linear relationship between CT number and physical density in units of g/cm^3.

A number of investigators have examined the errors inherent in a linear scaling of linear attenuation coefficients to values appropriate for gamma rays and megavoltage x rays used in radiation therapy. W. H. Payne and co-workers [25] and P. K. Kijewski and B. E. Bjarngard [17] have demonstrated that a linear scaling of the coefficients is satisfactory for all tissues except bone and that the presence of bone in the tissue cross-section can be flagged, and a separate correction factor applied. With a linear scaling factor, attenuation coefficients for sections of tissue through the region of interest can be computed for high-energy photons used in radiotherapy. A similar scaling process should be satisfactory for the design of treatment plans for electron therapy. For other modalities of radiation therapy (e.g., pions, alphas), the use of direct calibration techniques probably is preferable for converting CT numbers to parameters such as stopping powers which are used to estimate dose distributions [6, 14].

An alternative approach to determining attenuation coefficients appropriate to high-energy radiation therapy is CT with sources of radiation similar in energy to those employed therapeutically. Satisfactory sources include cobalt-60 and cesium-137, and a few investigators have explored the possibility of a high-energy CT unit dedicated to radiation-therapy treatment planning [1, 9, 26, 34]. The contrast and spatial resolution of these devices are severely limited compared to those of conventional CT units, and their practicality in clinical radiation therapy is not promising.

INHOMOGENEITY CORRECTIONS

From cross-sectional matrices of tissue characteristics such as attenuation coefficients, electron densities, stopping power ratios, and other parameters, corrections to the dose distribution can be computed for the presence of inhomogeneities such as lung and bone in the treatment fields [30]. However, commercial treatment-planning computers provide software packages for inhomogeneity corrections that correct only for the primary component of the radiation beam; that is, corrections are not made for the influence of inhomogeneities on the amount of scattered radiation reaching the tissues of interest. This neglect of scattered radiation can lead to significant errors in the dose distribution. Techniques for compensating for the effect of large inhomogeneities (e.g., the lungs) on the amount of radiation scattered to a region of interest have been proposed by M. R. Sontag and J. R. Cunningham [31, 32]. Corrections for the influence of inhomogeneities on the dose distributions for electrons, pions, and heavy charged particles are being developed [3, 4, 6, 12, 21, 33].

DESIGN OF THE CT TREATMENT-PLANNING SYSTEM

Requirements of a CT unit for treatment planning in radiation therapy have been described by J. R. Stewart and co-workers [33]. Among these requirements are the following:

1. The patient should be positioned in an identical configuration for CT examination and for treatment. For example, the patient couch of the CT unit should resemble the treatment couch for the therapy unit [2].
2. The region scanned with the CT unit must be identifiable when the patient is positioned for treatment [18].
3. If numerical CT data are used by a treatment-planning computer, the format of the CT data should be compatible with the computer.
4. CT data should be presentable in any section desired through the region of interest.
5. CT numbers of water and air should be reproducible to within 2 percent, and the numbers should be linear to within 2 percent

over the range of materials of biological interest, excluding bone. In addition, the numbers should be uniform to within 2 percent over the central 90 percent of the image of a 30-cm-diameter water phantom [22, 23, 36].

6. A life-size print of the CT image should be available.
7. CT data should be easily convertible to attenuation coefficients normalized to water for the radiation to be used for treatment.

Various approaches can be taken to the use of CT in the design of treatment plans for radiation therapy. The simplest approach is optical magnification of the CT image to life size, and use of a tracing device such as a (ρ-θ) plotter to enter information such as patient contour, outline of critical organs, and tumor location into the treatment-planning computer. Inhomogeneities are described by average densities, expressed either as representative values for the structures or as values obtained by averaging CT numbers over appropriate regions in the image. This approach has certain limitations but does permit use of CT for treatment planning when data from the CT unit cannot be entered directly into the treatment-planning computer. One limitation is the spatial distortion in patient anatomy that may occur during optical magnification of the CT image [15]. Other limitations of this approach include the unavailability of isodose distributions superimposed on CT images and the inability to use individual CT numbers for inhomogeneity corrections.

For direct utilization of CT data in treatment planning, at least three methods are possible. In the first, an interface is provided to transfer data between the CT unit and the treatment planning computer. Interfaces of this type are available from a number of manufacturers of treatment-planning computer systems. A second method uses the CT computer as a treatment-planning computer. Most manufacturers of CT units offer treatment-planning packages as an option at extra cost. A third method is development of CT units especially designed for data acquisition and treatment planning in radiation therapy. Each of these methods offers the opportunity to improve treatment planning in radiation therapy. A particular method should be selected only after careful review of each approach and its compatibility with the facilities and resources available to the user [7, 8, 13, 16].

REFERENCES

1. Battista, J. J., and Bronskill, M. J. Compton-scatter tissue densitometry: Calculation of single- and multiple-scatter photon fluences. *Phys. Med. Biol.* 23:1, 1978.

2. Battista, J. J., Rider, W. D., and Van Dyk, J. Computed tomography for radiotherapy planning. *Int. J. Radiat. Oncol. Biol. Phys.* 6:99, 1980.

3. Belgam, R. A., Cacak, R. K., and Hendee, W. R. Perturbations in electron ionization induced by inhomogeneities (abstract). *Med. Phys.* 8:564, 1981.

4. Berardo, P. A., and Zink, S. M. CT data and pion treatment planning at Los Alamos (abstract). *Med. Phys.* 5:326, 1978.

5. Brizel, H. E., Livingston, P. A., and Grayson, E. V. Radiotherapeutic application of pelvic computed tomography. *J. Comput. Assist. Tomogr.* 3:453, 1979.

6. Chen, G. T. Y., et al. Treatment planning for heavy-ion radiotherapy. *Int. J. Radiat. Oncol. Biol. Phys.* 5:1809, 1979.

7. Coffey, II, C. W. CT-assisted treatment-planning systems in radiotherapy. Comparison of conventional and CT-assisted systems. I. *Appl. Radiol.* 10:55, 1981; II. *Appl. Radiol.* 10:109, 1981.

8. Edwards, M., et al. A computed tomography–radiation therapy treatment-planning system utilizing a whole-body CT scanner. *Med. Phys.* 8:242, 1981.

9. Friedman, M. I., Beattie, J. W., and Laughlin, J. S. Cross-sectional absorption density reconstruction for treatment planning. *Phys. Med. Biol.* 19:819, 1974.

10. Geise, R. A., and McCullough, E. C. The use of CT scanners in megavoltage photon-beam therapy planning. *Radiology* 124:133, 1977.

11. Goitein, M., et al. The value of CT scanning in radiation therapy treatment planning: A prospective study. *Int. J. Radiat. Oncol. Biol. Phys.* 5:1787, 1979.

12. Goitein, M. The measurement of tissue heterodensity to guide charged-particle radiotherapy. *Int. J. Radiat. Oncol. Biol. Phys.* 3:27, 1977.

13. Goitein, M. Computed tomography in planning radiation therapy. *Int. J. Radiat. Oncol. Biol. Phys.* 5:445, 1979.

14. Hills, J., Hendee, W. R., and Smith, A. Converting CT numbers to stopping powers for pion therapy treatment planning (abstract). *Med. Phys.* 5:325, 1978.

15. Ibbott, G. S. Radiation therapy treatment planning and the distortion of CT images. *Med. Phys.* 7:261, 1980.

16. Kelsey, C. A., et al. CT scanner selection and specification for radiation therapy. *Med. Phys.* 7:555, 1980.

17. Kijewski, P. K., and Bjarngard, B. E. The use of computed tomography data for radiotherapy dose calculations. *Int. J. Radiat. Oncol. Biol. Phys.* 4:429, 1978.

18. Kubota, K., et al. Some devices for computed tomography radiotherapy treatment planning. *J. Comput. Assist. Tomogr.* 4:697, 1980.

19. MacDonald, J. S., et al. Changes in patient treatment arising from CT scanning. Presented at the 63rd Annual Meeting, Radiological Society of North America, Chicago, 1977.

20. McCullough, E. C. Computed Tomography in Radiation Therapy Treatment Planning. In T. H. Newton and D. G. Potts (eds.), *Radiology of the Skull and Brain: Technical Aspects of Computed Tomography.* St. Louis: Mosby, 1981. P. 4301.

21. McCullough, E. C. Potentials of computed tomography in radiation therapy treatment planning. *Radiology* 129:765, 1978.

22. McCullough, E. C., et al. Performance evaluation and quality assurance of computed tomography scanners, with illustrations from the EMI, ACTA, and DELTA scanners. *Radiology* 120:173, 1976.

23. McCullough, E. C., and Krueger, A. M. Performance evaluation of computerized treatment

planning systems for radiotherapy: External photon beams. *Int. J. Radiat. Oncol. Biol. Phys.* 6:1599, 1980.

24. Munzenrider, J. E., et al. Use of body scanner in radiotherapy treatment planning. *Cancer* 40:170, 1977.

25. Payne, W. H., et al. Extrapolation of linear attenuation coefficients of biologic materials from diagnostic-energy x-ray levels to the megavoltage range. *Med. Phys.* 4:505, 1977.

26. Payne, W. H., et al. Treatment planning in cobalt-60 radiotherapy using computerized tomography techniques. *Med. Phys.* 5:48, 1978.

27. Phelps, M. E., Gado, M. H., and Hoffman, E. J. Correlation of effective atomic number and electron density with attenuation coefficients measured with polychromatic x rays. *Radiology* 117:585, 1975.

28. Prasad, S. C., Glasgow, G. P., and Purdy, J. A. Dosimetric evaluation of a computed tomography treatment-planning system. *Radiology* 130:777, 1979.

29. Ragan, D. P., and Perez, C. A. Efficacy of CT-assisted two-dimensional treatment planning: Analysis of 45 patients. *AJR* 131:75, 1978.

30. Sontag, M. R., et al. Implications of computed tomography for inhomogeneity corrections in photon-beam dose calculations. *Radiology* 124:143, 1977.

31. Sontag, M. R., and Cunningham, J. R. Corrections to absorbed dose calculations for tissue inhomogeneities. *Med. Phys.* 4:431, 1977.

32. Sontag, M. R., and Cunningham, J. R. The equivalent tissue-air ratio method for making absorbed dose calculations in heterogeneous medium. *Radiology* 129:787, 1978.

33. Stewart, J. R., et al. Computed tomography in radiation therapy. *Int. J. Radiat. Oncol. Biol. Phys.* 4:313, 1978.

34. Thieme, G. A., et al. Cross-sectional anatomic images by gamma-ray transmission scanning. *Acta Radiol. Oncol. Radiat. Phys. Biol.* 14:81, 1975.

35. Van Houtte, P., et al. Computed axial tomography (CAT) contribution for dosimetry and treatment evaluation in lung cancer. *Int. J. Radiat. Oncol. Biol. Phys.* 6:995, 1980.

36. White, D. R., Speller, R. D., and Taylor, P. M. Evaluating performance characteristics in computerized tomography. *Br. J. Radiol.* 54:221, 1981.

13   Advances in X-Ray Computed Tomography

Transmission computed tomography (CT) has made major advances over a relatively short period, as is exemplified by the four generations of CT scanners that have evolved over the first ten years of commercial development of CT units. These advances primarily reflect improvements in the mechanical design of CT units that have yielded improvements in resolution and have resulted in faster imaging times. As the units have utilized an increasingly simple motion (e.g., purely circular motion of detectors, x-ray source, or both, the rate of evolution of CT units has decreased. Although future improvements in transmission CT probably will occur at a slower pace, there is little reason to doubt that they will occur.

There are four fundamental characteristics of CT units that might be expected to improve in future scanners. These characteristics are volume imaging, and spatial, contrast, and temporal resolution. Each of these characteristics, with its potential for improvement, is discussed in the following sections.

VOLUME IMAGING

Current CT units provide images of multiple transverse tomographic sections through the region of interest in the patient. With most units, data in different sections can be combined by software techniques to furnish longitudinal (e.g., coronal and sagittal) and oblique images of patient anatomy, usually with an accompanying reduction in spatial resolution. The simultaneous accumulation of transmission data for a three-dimensional block of tissue is an objective being pursued by a few investigators at the present time. Realization of this objective would permit the display of images oriented at any desired angle through the block of tissue.

In present CT units, the spatial resolution along the body axis is determined by the width of the x-ray beam and is far inferior to that in a transverse plane. With a three-dimensional block of projection data (consisting, for example, of $512 \times 512 \times 512$ volume elements, each $1 \times 1 \times 1$ mm in size), the spatial resolution could be improved significantly along the body axis, and the presence of partial volume and misregistration artifacts could be reduced in the resulting images.

To produce a three-dimensional block of CT numbers rather than a sequence of essentially two-dimensional sections of CT numbers, an x-ray beam shaped like a cone is used. In addition, a two-dimensional array of detectors is required in place of the one-dimensional matrix employed currently. The cone-shaped x-ray beam and the area detector array are rotated about the patient in a fashion similar to that employed in a conventional third-generation CT unit. In this approach, anatomic regions near the edge of the x-ray beam are not exposed to x rays during all orientations of the x-ray beam. These regions of limited sampling create problems during image reconstruction. The problems can be reduced by employing more than one x-ray source for the transmission measurements [17].

Transmission data measured for a rotating, cone-shaped x-ray beam and matrix of radiation detectors require rather sophisticated techniques to accomplish image reconstruction in a reasonable period of time. To simplify the reconstruction process, cone-beam units that scan linearly at certain angular orientations have been proposed [2]. Problems of incomplete collection of projection data and reduced efficiency of x-ray detection have limited the interest in this approach to volume scanning in CT.

For the two-dimensional detector required for cone-beam scanning, several approaches have been proposed. For example, N. A. Baily [1] has digitized the signal from an image-intensifier television system in the manner employed today in digital fluoroscopy. An alternative approach involves the use of solid-state detectors such as cesium iodide, bismuth germanate, and cadmium tungstate coupled to light-sensitive photodiodes. Other solid-state detectors under investigation include cadmium telluride, mercuric iodide, and high-purity germanium [2].

One of the advantages of CT is its superior rendition of low-contrast information. This superior rendition is due in part to the small amount of scattered radiation present in single-section CT compared to conventional roentgenographic techniques. This advantage is compromised in volume-imaging CT employing cone-shaped x-ray beams, because scattered radiation increases with the area of the x-ray beam. To eliminate scattered radiation, a grid arrangement probably will be required in front of the radiation detectors used for volume imaging. In addition, some reduction in the effects of scattered radiation may be achievable with software filtering techniques.

SPATIAL RESOLUTION

Improvements in spatial resolution to values below 1 mm are being sought by most manufacturers of CT units. However, these improvements usually are realized at the expense of increased image noise, because reductions in the size of the volume elements required to improve spatial resolution result in sampling the volume elements with fewer x rays. The increased noise of the resultant images leads to a reduction in contrast resolution. To maintain the noise level, and therefore the contrast resolution, at an acceptable level, longer imaging times are necessary. However, longer imaging times degrade the temporal resolution. Because contrast and temporal resolution are probably more important than spatial resolution in obtaining clinically significant information in CT, an emphasis on improving spatial resolution probably is unwise, even though this emphasis exists with some manufacturers of CT units. The only apparent solution to this quandary appears to be the design of x-ray tubes with a higher capacity to generate x rays. A few manufacturers of x-ray tubes are supporting major research efforts to accomplish this objective.

CONTRAST RESOLUTION

The term *contrast resolution* describes the ability of an x-ray imaging system to distinguish subtle differences in the composition of tissues from one region of anatomy to the next. The importance of contrast resolution in revealing clinically useful information about the patient has been accentuated significantly by the advent of CT, and contrast resolution is now recognized as at least equal in importance to spatial resolution in the visualization of disease in many patients.

Contrast resolution is limited primarily by image noise in most imaging systems, including transmission CT. Noise in an image arises from a variety of sources, including the x-ray tube (quantum mottle), the patient (tissue structure noise), the radiation detectors (receptor noise), the reconstruction program (reconstruction noise), and the display system (display noise). The first two of these sources of image noise usually are the most significant, and they are discussed here.

The term *quantum mottle* describes the imprecision in CT numbers caused by the limited number of x rays used for each of the measurements of x-ray transmission. This contribution to image noise increases with a reduction in the number of x rays accompanying, for example, a decrease in the size of individual volume elements. In transmission CT, quantum mottle often is the major contributor to image noise and, consequently, is frequently the major limitation in the contrast resolution available in the image. Quantum mottle can be reduced only by using

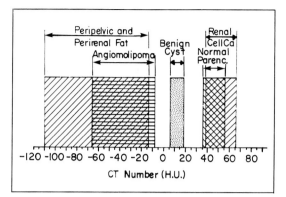

FIGURE 13-1.   *Overlap of CT numbers for selected body constituents. (Reprinted from R. S. Pickering, et al. Computed tomography of the excised kidney.* Radiology *113:643, 1974. With permission.)*

more x rays for the transmission measurements, and it is responsible for the renewed interest in the design of x-ray tubes with high capacities for x-ray generation.

The term *tissue-structure noise* refers to variations in the x-ray attenuation properties of a specific type of tissue. In Table 13-1, for example, similarities in electron density are illustrated for different body tissues. Distinction of these different tissues in a CT image requires a rather sophisticated level of contrast resolution. The overlap of CT numbers for different tissues is illustrated in Figure 13-1 for one type of CT unit.

Because of the subtle differences in body composition that are of interest in a CT image, improvement of contrast resolution is a desirable objective in CT. In addition to reductions in quantum mottle being sought by the design of new x-ray tubes, other approaches to improving contrast resolution are being pursued. These approaches primarily involve the use of contrast agents to enhance differences in the x-ray transmission characteristics of various tissues. Improvements in the use of contrast agents are being sought along two separate pathways. These pathways are (1) subtraction techniques (temporal, energy) and (2) development of new contrast agents (improvement of physical properties and improvement of chemical properties).

Table 13-1.   *Electron Densities for Selected Body Constituents*

Constituent	Physical Density (kg/m^3)	Electron Density (electrons/kg)	Electron Density (electrons/m^3)
Air	1.29	3.01×10^{26}	3.88×10^{26}
Blood	1055	3.89×10^{26}	4.10×10^{29}
Bone	1650–1850	$3.00–3.19 \times 10^{26}$	5.42×10^{29}
Brain	1034		
Fat	910	$3.34–3.48 \times 10^{26}$	3.10×10^{29}
Kidney	1040	3.85×10^{26}	4.01×10^{29}
Muscle	1080	3.89×10^{26}	4.20×10^{29}
Water	1000	3.34×10^{26}	3.34×10^{29}

Subtraction Techniques

The visualization of subtle pathology in a CT image is impaired by the presence of significant amounts of nonessential information. By subtracting this nonessential "background" information from the image, the perception of clinically useful information can often be improved. Subtraction can be performed in either temporal or energy modes.

Temporal Subtraction. Temporal subtraction is performed by subtracting an earlier image from one made later of the same region, but after the administration of a contrast agent. In CT, the subtraction is performed pixel by pixel, so that all that is revealed in the subtraction image is the difference in the two images [16, 34]. If spatial alignment of the two images is perfect, the only difference revealed in the subtraction image ideally is the distribution of the contrast agent. In practice, this approach is subject to several problems. For example, small amounts of patient motion can create registration errors that cause incomplete subtraction of information common to the preenhanced and postenhanced images. Also, beam hardening by the contrast agent in the postenhanced scan creates differences in the CT numbers for anatomy common to the two images. Of major consequence is the significant level of image noise in the subtraction image created when one relatively noisy image is subtracted from another.

Energy Subtraction. A second approach to the formation of subtraction images in CT is the technique of energy subtraction. In this approach, CT data are obtained with x-ray beams of two or more effective energies, and the data are weighted and subtracted to yield a subtraction image [14, 33]. The subtraction image reveals differences in the tissues that cause changes in the transmission of the x-ray beams. When iodinated contrast agents are present in the tissues, the effective x-ray energies often are positioned slightly above and below the k absorption edge of iodine, and the subtraction image reveals the distribution of iodine with a reasonable degree of clarity. This technique is called *k-edge subtraction* [24]. Even without contrast agents, energy-subtraction techniques sometimes are helpful, especially if the effective energies of the x-ray beams are sufficiently different (e.g., 100 kVp and 140 kVp). Compared to temporal subtraction methods, energy-subtraction techniques tend to produce noisier images and are somewhat less capable of revealing subtle differences in adjacent tissues [5].

In some applications of the energy-subtraction technique, two or more images are obtained sequentially, with the kVp of the x-ray beam changed between successive images. This approach is subject to the misregistration errors discussed above for temporal subtraction. A preferred approach is to obtain the information for both images essentially simultaneously, with the kVp across the x-ray tube alternating from one value to the other between successive x-ray pulses. This technique reduces problems of patient motion and misregistration of data. A third approach, pioneered by R. A. Brooks and G. Di Chiro [3], G. L. Brownell [4], and A. Fenster [8], involves the use of a single-energy x-ray beam with two or more "split" detectors that receive the transmitted x-ray beam after it has passed through different amounts of filtration. After weighting the signals from the different detectors to compensate for differences in intensity, the signals are subtracted to yield a difference image similar to that obtained with x-ray beams of different effective energies.

Different approaches to multiple energy-subtraction imaging are illustrated in Figure 13-2.

Development of New Contrast Agents

Contrast agents can be improved in at least two ways: (1) by selection of contrast materials with improved physical properties that lead to in-

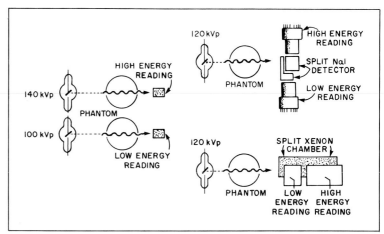

FIGURE 13-2. *Methods of multiple energy subtraction imaging in computed tomography.* Left: *Dual-kVp technique.* Right: *Split-detector approach using either scintillation detectors* (top) *or ionization chambers* (bottom). *(Reprinted from D. B. Plewes, M. R. Violante, and T. W. Morris, Intravenous Contrast Material and Tissue Enhancement in Computed Tomography. In G. D. Fullerton and J. A. Zagzebski {eds.}, Medi-*cal Physics of CT and Ultrasound: Tissue Imaging and Characterization. *New York: American Institute of Physics, 1980. P. 176. With permission.)*

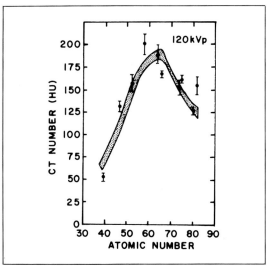

FIGURE 13-3.   *Variation in CT number (i.e., x-ray attenuation) as a function of absorber Z for a typical 120 kVp x-ray beam used in CT. Absorber is present at a concentration of 5 mg/μl. (Reprinted from D. B. Plewes, M. R. Violante, and T. W. Morris, Intravenous Contrast Material and Tissue Enhancement in Computed Tomography. In G. D. Fullerton and J. A. Zagzebski {eds.},* Medical Physics of CT and Ultrasound: Tissue Imaging and Characterization. *New York: American Institute of Physics, 1980. P. 176. With permission. Graph adapted from S. E. Seltzer, et al. Absorption of polychromatic x rays in a CT scanner by elements of high atomic number: Implications for development of improved contrast agents. Presented at the 27th AUR meeting, Rochester, N.Y., May 1979.)*

creased attenuation of x rays in the diagnostic energy range, and (2) by development of agents with chemical properties that yield improved differential uptake among the tissues of interest.

When low-energy x rays interact with materials of relatively high atomic number (Z), most interactions occur by the photoelectric process (Chapter 2). In general, the likelihood of photoelectric interactions decreases rapidly with increasing photon energy $h\nu$, varying approximately as $1/(h\nu)^3$. However, for materials such as iodine in the intermediate range of atomic numbers, higher-energy x rays are above the k absorption edge and are more likely to be absorbed. For any particular x-ray beam, there is an ideal atomic number for the absorbing material that yields a maximum absorption of the x-ray beam as a result of the energy of its k edge. For a typical x-ray beam used in CT, the range of atomic numbers for an ideal contrast agent is shown in Figure 13-3. These data reveal that elements with atomic numbers between about 58 and 62 provide the maximum difference in attenuation between tissue and the contrast agent. It is also apparent that iodine, with a Z of 53, is not far from this ideal range, and that the modest advantage of agents with slightly greater atomic numbers may not justify the extensive effort required for their development as contrast agents.

There are at least three possibilities for improving the pharmacologic behavior of contrast agents to yield more satisfactory contrast resolution. These possibilities lie in developing agents that (1) are site-specific in the sense that they concentrate primarily in diseased tissue and not in normal tissue, (2) are site-specific in the sense that they concentrate primarily in normal tissue and not in diseased tissue, and (3) are gaseous and exhibit relatively high solubilities in selected tissues. Each of these possibilities is discussed below.

Attempts to identify agents that concentrate only in lesions or other types of diseased tissue have proved relatively unsuccessful to date. One possibility is a solution of polyvinylpyrrolidone and metallic salts that has been shown to concentrate selectively in thigh abscesses in rabbits [32]. The mechanism of this retention is poorly understood, and efforts currently are under way to reproduce the results with metallic salts that are less toxic [22].

Materials that concentrate in normal, but not in diseased, tissues include selected agents that are removed from the bloodstream by phagocytic cells in the reticuloendothelial system of the liver and spleen. The first substance identified with this property was Thorotrast, a suspension of thorium oxide particles. Thorotrast was used for over 20 years in diagnostic radiology, but its use was discontinued after recognition of the high radiation doses delivered to the liver by the radioactive thorium [27]. Other inorganic compounds have been identified with properties similar to those of Thorotrast but without radioactive components; they have not been used clinically because they are retained indefinitely in the liver [9, 22].

Organic compounds exhibit shorter retention times in the reticuloendothelial system, and various substances that concentrate in normal tissues have been investigated for possible development as contrast agents. Among these compounds are water-insoluble ethyl esters of iothalamate and iodipamide [30], and oily emulsions of ethiodol [18, 19, 21, 29]. None of these compounds has been introduced into routine clinical use.

Several investigators have explored the potential of xenon as a contrast agent for brain imaging [6, 7, 11, 16, 20, 23, 31, 35]. Xenon is highly soluble in water and fatty tissue, and crosses the blood-brain barrier to diffuse into brain tissue. It is about twice as soluble in gray matter as in white matter because of the greater lipid content of gray matter. Xenon appears to be soluble to different degrees in various brain tumors. The relative concentration of xenon in a particular tumor depends not only on these relative solubilities but also on the rate of flow of blood to the tumor, since the xenon is carried to the tumor in dissolved form in the blood.

TEMPORAL RESOLUTION

Over the first few years of development of CT units, dramatic improvements in scan time (temporal resolution) were achieved. These improvements are illustrated in Figure 3-1; they reflect simplifications in scanner geometry from a translate-rotate to a purely rotational motion. Today, most CT units require times as short as two seconds for accumulation of transmission data during a complete 360-degree rotation of the CT gantry. Some manufacturers have recently offered even shorter scan times by providing software that permits the reconstruction of images from transmission data accumulated over a partial rotation of the CT gantry. The zone of segmented reconstruction can be shifted during the scanning process so that a series of successive images is provided, with data for each image obtained in times on the order of a second or so. Because these images are reconstructed from data obtained during a partial, rather than a complete, rotation, they tend to exhibit reduced spatial resolution and frequent artifacts. Particularly troublesome are streak artifacts caused by boluses of contrast agents that change in position from one partial scan to the next. Nevertheless, partial-scan images are useful in studying rapidly changing processes in the body. In particular, this approach to CT imaging, usually referred to as *dynamic scanning*, is helpful in studying rapid changes in the distribution of a contrast agent [12, 13, 28]. Capabilities of selected CT manufacturers to offer dynamic scanning are described in Table 13-2. The number of dynamic scans that can be performed successively usually is limited by the heat capacity of the x-ray tube.

Of particular interest is the use of CT to pro-

Table 13-2.   *Dynamic Scanning Capabilities of Selected CT Units*

CT Unit	Model	Scan Time (sec)	Reset Time (sec)	Total Cycle Time (sec)	Max. No. of Successive Scans	No. of Scans Limited By	Images Per Scan	Time Span Single Image (sec)	Physiologic Gating
Elscint	1002	1.8	0.7	2.5	35 +	Computer storage	1	1.8	
	2002	1.8	0.7	2.5	35 +	Computer storage			Under development
General Electric	8800	4.8	1.4	6.2	15	X-ray tube	Up to 3	2.8	Under development
	9800	2.0	2.5	4.5	20	X-ray tube			Under development
Interad	Whole body	3.0	1.5	4.5	150	Computer storage	Up to 7	1.5	
Omnimedical	Quad I	1.5	1.5	3.0	4 + 4	Computer storage	1	1.5	
Philips	Tomoscan 310	4.8	1.1	5.9	15	Computer storage	4	1.2	Under development (available mid-1982)
Picker	Synerview 600	1.7	0.8	2.5	10–12	X-ray tube	Typically 6 (up to 300)	0.85	Manual gating
	Synerview 1200	1.7	0.8	2.5	10–15	X-ray tube	6 (600)	0.85	Manual gating
Siemens	DR2	3.2	1.8	5	60	X-ray tube	3	2.1	Available as option
	DR3	3.2	1.8	5	60	X-ray tube	3	2.1	Available as option
Technicare	2060	2.0	4.0 with dynamic option	6.0	15	X-ray tube	1	2.0	Under development (available mid-1982)
Toshiba	TCT-65A	4.5	2.0	6.5	12	X-ray tube	3	2.6	

duce essentially static images of the heart in times as short as 100 msec. Three approaches have been proposed for these images: (1) retrospective gating (post-scan data acquisition) with a conventional CT unit; (2) prospective gating (pre-scan data acquisition) with a conventional CT unit; and (3) scanning with a very fast CT unit designed specifically for cardiovascular studies. Each of the gating techniques involves the correlation of CT data acquisition or display with an electrocardiographic recording of the patient's heart cycle; each is limited by registration errors of the heart's position from one cardiac cycle to the next.

In *retrospective gating*, transmission data are collected over several rotations of the CT unit. For image reconstruction, only those data are used that were collected during successive intervals of the desired phase of the cardiac cycle as determined from the electrocardiographic recording. In Figure 13-4, for example, the image is reconstructed from data collected during only a portion (segments 3 and 4) of the cardiac cycle. A major advantage of retrospective gating is that transmission data for the entire cardiac cycle are available for selective use during the image-reconstruction process.

Prospective gating is similar to retrospective gating except that data are collected only during the period of interest in the cardiac cycle. X-ray transmission data are not collected during other phases of the cycle and are not available for image reconstruction should this be desired later. The major advantages of prospective gating are reduced loading of the x-ray tube and reduced radiation dose to the patient. An example of prospective gating of x-ray transmission data in correlation with the cardiac cycle is shown in the bottom line of Figure 13-4.

To improve the temporal resolution of CT units for accumulation of transmission data over 360 degrees of rotation, modifications of the present design of CT units are necessary. These modifications are required because x-ray tubes are not designed mechanically to withstand the stress of rotating 360 degrees in times as short as a few hundred milliseconds. To achieve imaging times of 100 to 200 msec, more than a single x-ray tube is required as the source of x rays. Several investigators are attempting to develop an ultra-fast CT unit with scan times of 100 msec or less. This development requires the use of multiple x-ray sources, either as discrete x-ray tubes in a ring configuration around the patient or as a continuous x-ray source produced by scanning an electron beam around a circular anode surrounding the patient.

The first approach is the principle of the "dynamic spatial reconstructor" (DSR) under development at the Mayo Clinic [25, 26]. In this device, 28 separate x-ray tubes are aligned with 28 light amplifier–television chains positioned behind a single fluorescent screen on the opposite side of the patient (see Figure 3-10). This apparatus rotates around the body at a speed of 15 revolutions per minute to yield a new set of 28 two-dimensional projections of x-ray transmission data every $\frac{1}{60}$ second. The actual scan time for the 28 projections is about 10 msec, with each x-ray tube pulsed for about 0.34 msec during the scan. Up to 240 adjacent tomographic sections, each 1 mm thick, can be imaged for each set of 28 projections. The radiation exposure to the patient is about 20 mR for each set of 28 projections. Limitations of the DSR include its high cost and possible restrictions in the degree of contrast resolution attainable. The hardware assembly for the DSR is illustrated in Figure 13-5.

An alternative approach to rapid CT imaging involves the use of a circular x-ray anode and an electron beam that is deflected magnetically to sweep around the ring-like anode. This approach was proposed by T. A. Iinuma and co-workers [15] and J. Haimson [10] and is used in the cardiovascular CT (CVCT) unit being developed by D. P. Boyd [2]. In the CVCT, the electron beam is scanned both along and trans-

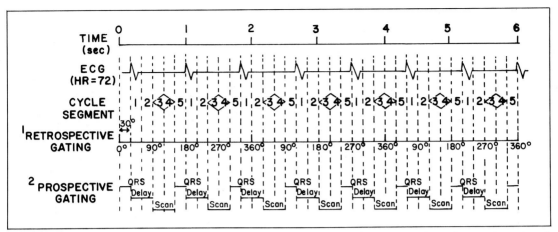

FIGURE 13-4. *Retrospective and prospective gating of x-ray transmission data in correlation with the cardiac cycle. (Reprinted from R. A. Robb, et al. The DSR: A high-speed three-dimensional x-ray computed tomography system for dynamic spatial reconstruction of the heart and circulation.* IEEE Trans. Nucl. Sci. *NS-26:2713, 1979. With permission.)*

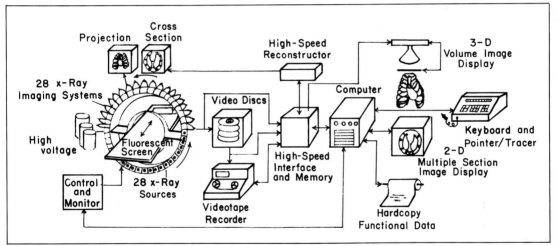

FIGURE 13-5. *Major components of the Dynamic Spatial Reconstructor. (Reprinted from R. A. Robb, A. H. Lent, and A. Chu.* Proc. 13 HICSS *3:384, 1980. With permission.)*

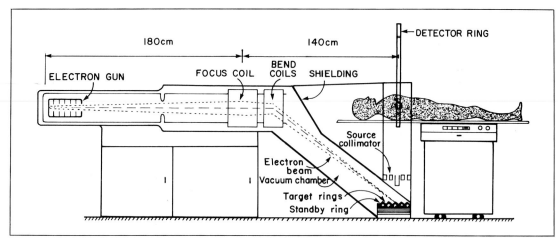

FIGURE 13-6. *Cross-sectional view of the CVCT scanner. (Reprinted from D. P. Boyd, Transmission Computed Tomography. In T. H. Newton and D. G. Potts {eds.},* Radiology of the Skull and Brain: Technical Aspects of Computed Tomography. *St. Louis: Mosby, 1981. P. 4357. With permission.)*

verse to the anode ring to create an area source of x rays that is viewed by a ring of 210 scintillation detectors. The x-ray beam is shaped like an inverted cone, with the base of the cone at the anode and the apex at the detectors (Figure 13-6). The inverted-cone geometry for the x-ray beam reduces the number of detectors required for measurement of x-ray transmission, but it requires extremely fast detectors for data acquisition. By combining four separate x-ray anodes with two independent detector rings, eight tomographic sections, each 1 cm thick, can be obtained during four successive sweeps of the electron beam. Each sweep requires 25 msec and produces two images, so that eight tomographic images can be obtained in 100 msec. Although the spatial resolution and contrast resolution of the CVCT and the DSR units are expected to be inferior to those in conventional CT, the superior temporal resolution is a definite advantage, especially for the study of rapidly changing processes such as cardiac anatomy and the dynamic flow of contrast agents.

REFERENCES

1. Baily, N. A. Computerized tomography using video techniques. *Opt. Eng.* 16:23, 1977.
2. Boyd, D. P. Transmission Computed Tomography. In T. H. Newton and D. G. Potts (eds.), *Radiology of the Skull and Brain: Technical Aspects of Computed Tomography.* St. Louis: Mosby, 1981. P. 4357.
3. Brooks, R. A., and Di Chiro, G. Split-detector computed tomography: A preliminary report. *Radiology* 126:255, 1978.
4. Brownell, G. L. Energy-sensitive detection and imaging. International Symposium on Computed Tomography, Miami Beach, Fla., March, 1978.
5. Cohen, G., and DiBianca, F. A. The use of contrast-detail–dose evaluation of image quality in a computed tomographic scanner. *J. Comput. Assist. Tomogr.* 3:189, 1979.
6. Drayer, B. P., et al. Physiologic change in regional cerebral blood flow defined by xenon-enhanced CT scanning. *Neuroradiology* 16:220, 1978.

7. Drayer, B. P., et al. Experimental xenon enhancement with CT imaging: Cerebral applications. *AJR* 134:39, 1980.

8. Fenster, A. Split xenon detector for tomochemistry in computed tomography. *J. Comput. Assist. Tomogr.* 2:243, 1978.

9. Fischer, H. W., and Zimmerman, G. R. Long retention of stannic oxide. Lack of tissue reaction in laboratory animals. *Arch. Path.* 88:259, 1969.

10. Haimson, J. X-ray source without moving parts for ultra-high speed tomography. *IEEE Trans. Nucl. Sci.* NS-26:2857, 1979.

11. Haughton, V., et al. Clinical cerebral blood flow measurement with inhaled xenon and CT. *AJR* 134:281, 1980.

12. Heinz, E. R., et al. Dynamic computed tomography study of the brain. *J. Comput. Assist. Tomogr.* 3:641, 1979.

13. Heinz, E. R., et al. A preliminary investigation of the role of dynamic computed tomography in renovascular hypertension. *J. Comput. Assist. Tomogr.* 4:63, 1980.

14. Hounsfield, G. N. Computerized transverse axial scanning (tomography). I. Description of system. *Br. J. Radiol.* 46:1016, 1973.

15. Iinuma, T. A., et al. Proposed system for ultrafast computed tomography. *J. Comput. Assist. Tomogr.* 1:494, 1977.

16. Kelcz, F., et al. Computed tomographic measurement of the xenon brain-flood partition coefficient and implications for regional cerebral blood flow: A preliminary report. *Radiology* 127:385, 1978.

17. Kowalski, G. Multi-slice reconstruction from twin-cone beam scanning. *IEEE Trans. Nucl. Sci.* NS-26:2895, 1979.

18. Lamarque, J. L., et al. The use of iodolipids in hepatosplenic computed tomography. *J. Comput. Assist. Tomogr.* 3:21, 1979.

19. Laval-Jeantet, M., et al. Hepatosplenography by intravenous injection of a new iodized oily emulsion. *Acta Radiol. {Diagn.}* (Stockholm) 17:49, 1976.

20. O'Brien, M. D., and Veall, N. Partition coefficients between various brain tumours and blood for ^{133}Xe. *Phys. Med. Biol.* 19:472, 1974.

21. Pinet, A., et al. Hepatography with intravenously injected emulsified iodolipids: Preliminary results. *Acta Radiol. {Diagn.}* (Stockholm) 17:41, 1976.

22. Plewes, D. B., Violante, M. R., and Morris, T. W. Intravenous Contrast Material and Tissue Enhancement in Computed Tomography. In G. D. Fullerton and J. A. Zagzebski (eds.), *Medical Physics of CT and Ultrasound: Tissue Imaging and Characterization.* AAPM Monograph No. 6. New York: American Institute of Physics, 1980. P. 176.

23. Radue, E. W., and Kendall, B. E. Xenon enhancement in tumours and infarcts. *Neuroradiology* 16:224, 1978.

24. Reiderer, S., and Mistretta, C. A. Selective iodine imaging using k-edge energies in computerized x-ray tomography. *Med. Phys.* 4:474, 1977.

25. Robb, R. A., et al. The DSR: A high-speed three-dimensional x-ray computed tomography system for dynamic spatial reconstruction of the heart and circulation. *IEEE Trans. Nucl. Sci.* NS-26:2713, 1979.

26. Robb, R. A. High-Speed Three-Dimensional Computed Tomography and Multidimensional Display of the Heart, Lungs, and Circulation. In G. D. Fullerton and J. A. Zagzebski (eds.), *Medical Physics of CT and Ultrasound: Tissue Imaging and Characterization.* AAPM Monograph No. 6. New York: American Institute of Physics, 1980. P. 656.

27. Thomas, S. F., Henry, G. W., and Kaplan, H. S. Hepatolienography: Past, present, and future. *Radiology* 57:669, 1951.

28. Traupe, H., et al. Hyperfusion and enhancement in dynamic computed tomography of ischemic stroke patients. *J. Comput. Assist. Tomogr.* 3:627, 1979.

29. Vermess, M., et al. Development and experimental evaluation of a contrast medium for computed tomographic examination of the liver and spleen. *J. Comput. Assist. Tomogr.* 3:25, 1979.

30. Violante, M. R., et al. Particulate contrast media for computed tomographic scanning of the liver. *Invest. Radiol.* 15:S171, 1980.

31. Winkler, S. S., et al. Regional cerebral blood flow determination in transmission CT using stable xenon. International Symposium on Computed Tomography, Las Vegas, Nev., 1979.

32. Young, S. W., and Enzmann, D. Polyvinylpyrrolidone contrast enhancement: Abscess imaging. *Radiology* 133:511, 1979.

33. Zatz, L. M. Iodinated contrast media in cranial tomography. *Invest. Radiol.* 15:S155, 1980.

34. Zilkha, E., et al. Computer subtraction in regional cerebral blood-volume measurements using the EMI scanner. *Br. J. Radiol.* 49:330, 1976.
35. Zilkha, E., et al. Diagnosis of subdural hematoma by computed axial tomography: Use of xenon inhalation for contrast enhancement. *J. Neurol. Neurosurg. Psychiatry* 41:370, 1978.

14 Emission Computed Tomography

The principles of computed tomography (CT) are useful in medical imaging applications other than those that utilize transmitted x rays. In emission computed tomography (ECT), for example, tomographic images are reconstructed that reveal the distribution of a radioactive nuclide in the body. With this approach, image contrast and spatial resolution at depth can be improved compared to the contrast and resolution provided by conventional nuclear medicine procedures. In some ways, the reconstruction process is more difficult when the radiation is emitted from a radionuclide in the patient, because corrections are required for attenuation of the radiation through different thicknesses of tissue and for variations in distance between the detector and the radionuclide. Although these problems can be resolved in part by using positron-emitting radionuclides, most positron emitters require a cyclotron facility for their production. For these reasons, ECT has not evolved as rapidly as x-ray transmission CT, even though its clinical potential was initially explored well in advance of transmission techniques.

The earliest work on ECT was conducted by D. E. Kuhl, R. Q. Edwards, and co-workers at the University of Pennsylvania [21, 22]. These investigators used a rectilinear scanner that collected gamma-ray emission data as the detector moved tangentially across the patient at a number of angles. In addition to difficulties associated with the varying attenuation of radiation as a function of depth of the radionuclide within the patient, Kuhl and Edwards encountered other problems, such as the rather primitive state of computer software available for image reconstruction in the 1960s. For these and other reasons, ECT evolved slowly in its early years, and its contribution as an imaging modality is even today a subject of some speculation.

In the late 1960s, H. O. Anger attempted to produce analog tomographic images with the scintillation camera [1]. Anger's studies were followed by efforts of a number of investigators to obtain digital CT images with the scintillation camera [5, 18, 26]. These efforts, and the parallel work on positron-emission tomography, provided the foundation for the current status of ECT.

ECT is similar in principle to x-ray transmission CT. In transmission CT, x-ray attenuation properties are determined for a section of tissue through a patient, and these properties are depicted as a matrix of CT numbers for the tissue section. From the matrix of CT numbers, a gray-scale display can be generated to produce an image of the tissue section. The attenuation properties reflect differences in atomic number and physical density within the tissue section, and the resulting matrix of numbers or gray-scale display depicts the morphology of the section. ECT images depict the distribution of a radionuclide in one or more sections of tissue. Instead of section morphology, this distribution reflects physiologic processes that concentrate the radionuclide in one or more organs or body compartments. Data used to generate ECT images are distorted by the attenuating properties of tissues between the radionuclide and the surface of the body. These distortions in data must be corrected to make ECT images useful clinically; that is, the attenuation properties of tissue are exactly the information sought in transmission CT, whereas in ECT these properties distort the desired data and must be corrected for. These corrections make the image-reconstruction process more difficult in ECT.

In all approaches to ECT, techniques of image reconstruction follow certain general principles. First, count-rate profiles are obtained across one projection of the patient. These profiles can be obtained with a single detector that scans transversely across the patient, with multiple detectors in a linear configuration, or with a narrow region of interest extending across the area detector of a scintillation camera. Next, similar profiles are obtained with the detector or detectors at different angular orientations with respect to the patient. Each of these profiles is corrected for attenuation of photons in the patient (alternatively, attenuation corrections can be applied to the postprocessed reconstructed data), and the profile data are subjected to a reconstruction algorithm. In most applications, a convolution (filtered back-projection) algorithm is used for the reconstruction to furnish a matrix of data or an image representing the distribution of radioactivity in the tomographic tissue section of interest.

Several techniques have been developed to correct ECT data for the effects of photon attenuation [6]. Shown in Figure 14-1 are the effects of photon attenuation and their correction by the simple assumption that the attenuation coefficient remains constant throughout the tissue section of interest.

ECT offers an excellent opportunity to obtain quantitative data concerning the distribution of a radionuclide in a patient [15]. In addition, absolute measurements of the volume of organs or lesions can be obtained, provided that the thickness of the tissue section is known and that the boundaries of the organs or lesions can be determined [17, 19, 30]. With proper corrections for attenuation, the activity per unit volume (i.e., $\mu\text{Ci/cm}^3$) can be determined by ECT for a radionuclide distributed in vivo. This parameter is an excellent index for physiologic studies and for radiation dosimetry.

The subject of ECT can be separated into two topics, single-photon tomographic emission tomography and positron-emission tomography.

SINGLE-PHOTON EMISSION TOMOGRAPHY

In single-photon ECT (SPECT), radiopharmaceuticals may be used that are identical to

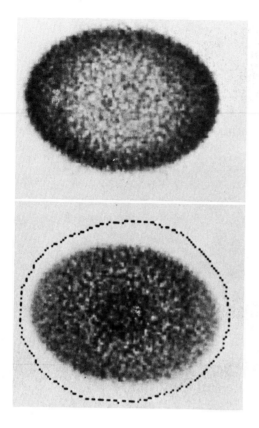

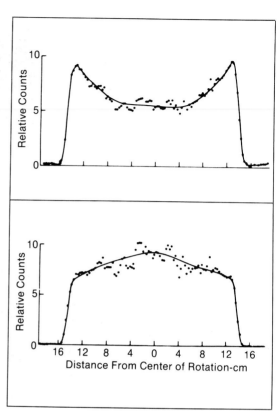

FIGURE 14-1.   Top: *Attenuation of 140 keV gamma rays from* ^{99m}Tc *is apparent in this transverse tomogram of a uniform 30- × 21-cm elliptical phantom.*
Bottom: *With the assumption that the attenuation coefficient remains constant throughout the phantom, a simple correction can be applied to reduce the variation in counts to ±10 percent along the major axis of the elliptical phantom. (Reprinted from P. H. Murphy, et al. Radionuclide computed tomography of the body using routine radiopharmaceuticals. I. System characterization. J. Nucl. Med. 20:102, 1979. With permission.)*

Table 14-1. *Single-Photon Tomographic Systems*

Longitudinal Type	Transaxial Type
Anger Pho-Con	Multicrystal
Coded Aperture	Rotating-Camera
Multiple-Pinhole	
Rotating Slant-Hole	

Source: Modified from P. N. Goodwin, Recent developments in
instrumentation for emission computed tomography. *Semin. Nucl.
Med.* 10:322, 1980.

those employed in conventional nuclear medicine imaging. Two approaches to SPECT have
been developed. In the first approach, termed
longitudinal tomography, images are formed in
planes parallel to the surface of the detectors.
The second approach (*transaxial tomography*) provides images perpendicular to the detector surfaces. With each of these approaches, image
contrast is improved in the tissue section of interest in the patient. Equipment for each of
these approaches is described in Table 14-1.

Longitudinal Tomography
The first commercial instrument to provide tomographic nuclear medicine images was developed by Searle Radiographics, Inc., from the
analog approach to tomography pioneered by
Anger [1]. This instrument, currently marketed
by Siemens Gammasonics under the trade name
Pho-Con, uses two scintillation detectors positioned on opposite sides of the patient. Each of
the detectors consists of a 9.3-in. diameter by
0.5-in.-thick sodium iodide crystal equipped
with 19 photomultiplier tubes and a focused
collimator. The detectors scan in synchrony
across the patient to accumulate gamma-ray
emission data used to form the tomographic image. Data for as many as 12 tomographic planes
spaced at selected intervals can be obtained from
one transverse scan, and computer programs are
available to produce transaxial as well as longitudinal images. One disadvantage of this approach to tomographic imaging is the cost relative to that with a conventional scintillation

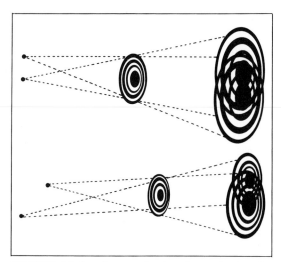

FIGURE 14-2. *In zone plate imaging, each point of radioactivity casts a unique shadow onto the detector. (Reprinted from M. H. Farmelant, et al. Initial clinical experiences with a Fresnel zone–plate imager. J. Nucl. Med. 16:183, 1975. With permission.)*

camera. Further information on the Pho-Con multiplanar tomographic imaging system is available in the literature [13].

A second approach to longitudinal tomography involves the use of coded apertures in place of the conventional collimators used with stationary scintillation cameras. This approach was pioneered by H. H. Barrett and colleagues [2], who used a Fresnel zone plate as a coded aperture. The Fresnel zone plate consists of a series of concentric lead rings separated by spaces transparent to gamma radiation. With the zone plate positioned between the scintillation camera and the patient, each point of radioactivity in the patient projects a unique image of the zone plate onto a film (Figure 14-2). When the processed film is illuminated by laser light (Figure 14-3), images are formed in longitudinal tomographic planes that vary in depth, depending on the distance of the viewer from the illuminated film. Compared to conventional collimators, zone-plate apertures are more sensitive because each point on the zone plate utilizes gamma rays from all, rather than just one, locations in the patient. However, the sensitivity is not uniform across the field of view of the collimator. In addition, zone-plate apertures yield a variety of image artifacts. Because of these problems, zone-plate apertures appear to have limited usefulness in clinical nuclear medicine. This limitation is particularly pronounced in the application of zone-plate apertures to imaging of larger regions of interest, because all parts of a large region contribute noise to the final image.

A modification of the zone-plate aperture approach to longitudinal tomographic imaging is the use of time-coded multiple apertures developed by W. L. Rogers and associates [27]. In the time-coded aperture approach, a lead plate containing a number of randomly positioned pinholes is stepped across a second plate fastened to the scintillation camera and containing evenly spaced multiple pinholes. The different

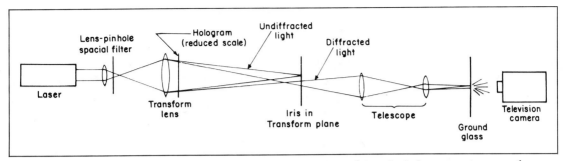

FIGURE 14-3.   *Optical reconstruction system for zone-plate imaging. (Reprinted from M. H. Farmelant, et al. Initial clinical experiences with a Fresnel zone–plate imager.* J. Nucl. Med. *16:183, 1975. With permission.)*

pinhole projections obtained at each step in the image-forming process constitute a set of projection data from which tomographic images can be reconstructed with separations as close as 1 cm. The point-source sensitivity of this technique is comparable to that provided by a high-sensitivity, parallel multihole collimator. However, the sensitivity decreases noticeably for an extended source.

The stationary multiple-pinhole technique for forming longitudinal tomographic images was developed in 1978 by Vogel and co-workers [29]. In earlier versions of this approach, a seven-pinhole collimator with lead dividers was positioned with the pinholes 12.7 cm from the scintillation crystal. The pinholes project seven separate images of the radioactivity distribution onto seven separate regions of the crystal. After correction for nonuniformity and spatial distortion, tomographic images can be produced from these projections by an iterative reconstruction process. Later versions of the technique have included expansion of the collimator to 12 pinholes and adaptation of the collimator to scintillation cameras with large fields of view. With the multiple-pinhole technique, all the projection data are obtained during a single exposure of about the same duration as that required for imaging with a conventional scintillation camera. Hence, motion artifacts are reduced in the image. Lateral resolution is reasonably satisfactory (7–10 mm full width at half maximum [FWHM] depending on depth). The major application of the multiple-pinhole technique has been in tomographic imaging of the heart. This application requires exact positioning of the heart under the pinhole collimator. The advantages of pinhole tomography are its low cost and the possibility of tomographic imaging with a conventional scintillation camera equipped with a pinhole collimator. The disadvantages include the rather small field of view and the poor depth resolution offered by this approach. Multiple-pinhole collimators and

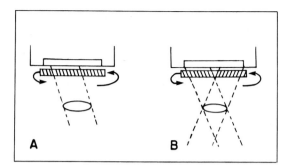

FIGURE 14-4. *Rotating slant-hole collimators for to-mographic nuclear medicine imaging. A. Rotating slant-hole collimator. B. Quadrant slant-hole collimator. (Reprinted from P. N. Goodwin, Recent developments in instrumentation for emission computed tomography. Semin. Nucl. Med. 10:322, 1980. With permission.)*

associated computer software are now offered by several companies as attachments to conventional scintillation cameras.

An alternative to the multiple-pinhole approach to tomographic imaging is use of rotating slant-hole collimators such as those described by G. Muehllehner in 1971 [23] (Figure 14-4A). An early version of the slant-hole collimator was marketed briefly by Nuclear Chicago (now Siemens Gammasonics) but did not achieve commercial viability. Employed in the collimator were multiple parallel holes, all slanted about 25 degrees from the vertical. During data acquisition the collimator rotated continuously below the crystal while the patient moved in a circular path. A similar approach, developed by G. S. Freedman, confined the acquisition of data to 12 specific orientations 30 degrees apart [11]. Both methods utilized analog techniques for image reconstruction.

More recent versions of slant-hole collimation for tomographic imaging have employed digital methods for image reconstruction. In these versions (e.g., the Tomovision system marketed by Technicare, Inc.) a rotating, 25-degree slant-hole collimator is mounted on a ring and rotated to six positions for data acquisition. From these six views, tomographic images parallel to the scintillation crystal are computed by iterative reconstruction techniques similar to those used for multiple-pinhole tomography. Up to 12 images can be produced at spacings of 1 to 2 cm between tomographic sections.

A modification of the parallel slant-hole approach to collimation is the quadrant slant-hole collimator developed by W. Chang, S. L. Lin, and R. E. Henkin [9, 10] (Figure 14-4B). In this technique, the collimator is divided into four sections, each with parallel holes slanting in a different direction with respect to the vertical. After four separate images have been obtained with this collimator, the device is rotated 45 degrees and four additional images are obtained. These eight projections are then recombined to form a reconstructed tomographic image.

Compared to stationary multiple-pinhole techniques, rotating slant-hole collimators offer a larger field of view, increased sensitivity, and improved lateral resolution at depth. Moreover, patient positioning is less critical. Disadvantages include their greater mechanical complexity and an inability to acquire all projection data simultaneously. The latter disadvantage reduces the usefulness of the method in dynamic studies. The rotating slant-hole collimator approach to tomographic imaging of the heart now appears as promising as the multiple-pinhole technique.

Transaxial Tomography

Single-photon transaxial tomography has evolved along two parallel paths. One path was initiated by Kuhl, Edwards, and colleagues [21, 22] and employs multiple detectors positioned in a specific geometry around the patient. The current version of this approach is designed exclusively for brain imaging and employs detectors on each side of a square with the patient's head at the center. To improve the spatial sampling of gamma-ray emission data, each detector is offset slightly to the side with respect to its counterpart on the opposite side of the patient. After multiple 50-sec rotations of the detectors around the patient, the gamma-ray emission data are combined to yield tomographic images.

Until 1980, a somewhat different multidetector tomographic scanner was marketed commercially by Union Carbide from a design developed by Cleon Corporation. In this instrument, named the *Cleon 710 Brain Imager,* 12 sodium iodide crystals with focused collimators are positioned around the patient. During a scan, each detector moves laterally while simultaneously moving in and out along a radius from the patient. At any moment, six crystals are moving toward the patient while the alternate six crystals are moving away. The entire array of

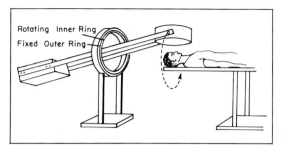

FIGURE 14-5. *The detector assembly and rotating gantry for the General Electric 400T scintillation camera. (Reprinted from P. N. Goodwin, Recent developments in instrumentation for emission computed tomography.* Semin. Nucl. Med. *10:322, 1980. With permission.)*

detectors rotates 18 degrees between successive lateral scans. A sequence of ten lateral scans requires 2 to 5 min, after which the patient table advances slightly and the scanning motions are repeated for the next tomographic section. Also marketed by Union Carbide was a Cleon 711 whole-body imaging system that employed ten sodium iodide crystals and furnished a larger field of view. Although the Union Carbide instruments are no longer available commercially, their ability to provide clinically useful information has been documented [12, 14].

Other multiple-crystal transaxial CT scanners for radionuclide imaging that have been marketed commercially include the Tomogscanner (J and P Engineering, Reading, England) and the Tomomatic 64, manufactured by Medimatic A/S, Denmark. All these multiple-crystal techniques for transaxial tomography require considerable time for image formation. This disadvantage ultimately may limit the clinical usefulness of this approach to transaxial tomography.

The second approach to transaxial tomography employs a single-crystal scintillation camera. In this approach, either the camera remains stationary and the patient rotates, or the camera rotates about a stationary patient. Because of patient discomfort associated with motion and the immobilization techniques required with a moving patient, the rotating-detector approach probably is preferable to the method requiring patient rotation. Early efforts to develop a rotating-camera system for CT include the work of J. W. Keyes, Jr. [20], and P. H. Murphy and co-workers [25].

The earliest rotating camera available commercially was the unit marketed by SELO Corporation of Milan. More recently, a rotating camera has been introduced by General Electric Company. This camera, termed the 400T, is mounted in a gantry so that the detector assembly can be rotated at any desired radius around the patient (Figure 14-5). Siemens Gammasonics and Picker International also have introduced a rotating-camera system for transaxial tomographic imaging. Among the advantages of a rotating camera for tomographic imaging are rapid image formation and its adaptability to conventional, as well as tomographic, imaging.

Relative evaluations of multiple-pinhole, rotating-collimator, multicrystal, and rotating-camera tomographic systems have begun to appear in the literature. The reader is referred to these publications for comparisons of imaging parameters such as resolution, sensitivity, and imaging times [7, 12, 14, 20, 25].

POSITRON-EMISSION TOMOGRAPHY

Interest has existed for many years in the formation of radionuclide images by detection of annihilation radiation released during positron decay of internally deposited radionuclides. This interest has been maintained primarily for two reasons:

First, the only readily available radioactive isotopes of oxygen, nitrogen, and carbon are the positron-emitting nuclides, ^{15}O, ^{13}N, and ^{11}C. These nuclides offer the opportunity for isotopic labeling of compounds of biological interest. Isotopic labeling provides labeled compounds that are more stable than those labeled nonisotopically with radioactive isotopes such as ^{99m}Tc and ^{131}I.

Second, the detection of annihilation radiation by coincidence-counting techniques eliminates the need for mechanical collimators. Deletion of the collimator significantly increases the number of photons available for image formation. Typically, as many as 50 percent of the annihilation photons escaping a region of interest are detected as coincidence events. This number represents an improvement in detection efficiency as high as tenfold compared to single-photon collimation. In addition, positron imaging provides automatic correction for the attenuation of photons in tissue between the detector and the radiation source.

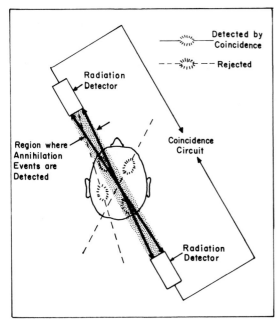

FIGURE 14-6.   *Electronic collimation available with positron-emitting radionuclides employs radiation detectors on opposite sides of the patient. The detectors operate in coincidence so that a signal is generated only when annihilation photons are absorbed simultaneously in both detectors. (Reprinted from M. Ter-Pogossian, The maturing of positron-emission tomography.* Diag. Imaging *3:26, 1981. With permission.)*

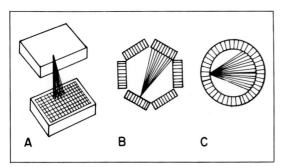

FIGURE 14-7.   *Three basic geometries for the detector assemblies of positron cameras. A. Parallel opposed detectors. B. Hexagonal arrays. C. Circular tomographic units composed of a single ring or multiple rings of detectors. (Reprinted from P. N. Goodwin, Recent developments in instrumentation for emission computed tomography.* Semin. Nucl. Med. *10:322, 1980. With permission.)*

Positron cameras (i.e., cameras that use annihilation radiation for image formation) have been under development in a few institutions for many years. Only relatively recently has this interest expanded to manufacturers of instruments for nuclear medicine imaging.

A number of radioactive nuclides decay by the emission of *positrons* (positively charged electrons that interact by ionization and excitation processes similar to those characteristic of ordinary electrons). In tissue, a positron travels a few millimeters while dissipating its energy by these interaction processes. The positron then combines with an electron, and the particles "annihilate," releasing two 0.51-MeV annihilation photons that leave the site of annihilation in opposite directions (i.e., at 180 degrees with respect to each other). It is this annihilation radiation that is imaged with a positron camera. If detectors on opposite sides of the patient are operated in coincidence, so that a signal is generated only when an annihilation photon is received by each detector, the origin of the annihilation photons and, therefore, the site of annihilation of the positron are known to be in the volume of tissue separating the two detectors. This site can be no more than a few millimeters from the origin of the positron and therefore from the location of the decaying atom. This approach to localization of the radioactive source is referred to as *electronic collimation;* it is inherently more sensitive, because mechanical collimators are eliminated. The principle of electronic collimation associated with the imaging of positron-emitting radionuclides is illustrated in Figure 14-6.

Three approaches to detector geometry have been followed in commercially available positron cameras. These approaches, classified as parallel-opposed multicrystal arrays, hexagonal arrays, and circular tomographic units, are outlined in Figure 14-7. Different techniques have been developed to provide multisection capability and adequate sampling of the emission of annihilation photons. Some of these techniques are described in Figure 14-8.

The design of positron cameras referred to as parallel-opposed multicrystal arrays was pioneered by G. L. Brownell and co-workers [4] at Massachusetts General Hospital. This design was incorporated into the PC4200 positron camera marketed for a time by the Cyclotron Corporation and described by L. R. Carroll [8]. The detector assembly consisted of opposing banks of 140 2- × 2-cm sodium iodide crystals arranged essentially as 12 × 12 arrays (less the corner crystals), with each crystal in one array operated in coincidence with a 5 × 5 matrix of crystals in the opposite array. In this manner, the detector assembly furnished 2,848 possible coincidence pairs of detectors. During a single scan, the detector assembly collected data at 29 angular positions to yield images of 23 separate tomographic sections spaced 1 to 4 cm apart.

The hexagonal-array approach to the design of detector assemblies for positron cameras was developed by M. M. Ter-Pogossian and colleagues [28]. The approach evolved through four stages, starting with PETT-I (positron-emission transaxial tomography) and ending with the PETT-IV tomographic unit. The PETT-III design was incorporated into a commercial unit known as the ECAT (emission computed axial tomography) marketed by EGG-ORTEX, Inc. This device is a single section positron-imaging system containing 66 sodium iodide crystals arranged as six banks of 11 crystals each. In a single bank, each detector is operated in coincidence with all 11 detectors in the opposite bank to yield 363 coincidence pairs of detectors. During a scan, each bank of detectors moves linearly for a distance of about 4 cm, and then rotates through 5-, 7.5-, or 10-degree angular increments over a total rotational arc of 60 degrees. Image resolution depends on the number of incremental steps in the linear and rotational motions, and it can be improved by detector collimation. The unit provides cardiac-gating

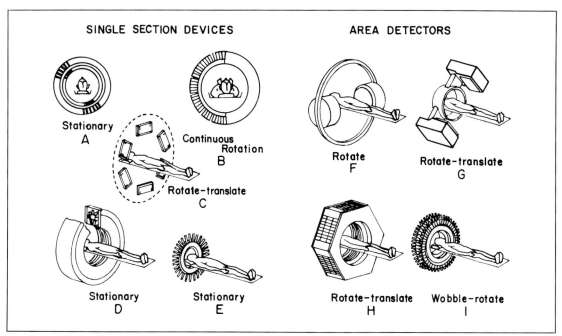

FIGURE 14-8. *Different detector arrangements for positron cameras to achieve multisection capability and adequate linear and angular sampling of emitted radiation. (Reprinted from M. Ter-Pogossian, The maturing of positron-emission tomography.* Diag. Imaging *3:26, 1981. With permission.)*

capability by using a buffer memory to partition data collected during different phases of the cardiac cycle.

Positron cameras consisting of one or more rings of scintillation detectors surrounding the patient appear to offer advantages over the alternative designs described above. Among these advantages are increased sensitivity per section and the capability of producing as many as nine tomographic sections simultaneously. The spatial resolution of ring-detector cameras currently is on the order of 7 to 8 mm, with some potential for improvement to values of 4 to 5 mm. However, the finite range of positrons in tissue and the angular divergence of the annihilation photons establish a resolution limit of several millimeters. Recent versions of the PETT scanner (PETT-V and -VI) have adopted the ring-detector design, as have several equipment manufacturers. For example, Atomic Energy of Canada Limited (AECL) has introduced the Therascan 3128, consisting of two rings of BGO detectors. This camera provides three image sections simultaneously, with the center slice produced by cross-coincidence between the rings. Bismuth germanate (BGO) detectors are used because the greater physical density of BGO compared to sodium iodide yields increased absorption of incident annihilation photons. Also, BGO exhibits reduced afterglow of the radiation-induced fluorescence, so that higher count rates can be obtained with BGO without significant coincidence count-rate loss. One disadvantage of BGO is that its fluorescence intensity (i.e., light output) is only about 10 percent that of sodium iodide. Another detector with some promise is cesium fluoride [24]. The fluorescence afterglow of this detector is very short (fluorescence decay time of 5 nsec).

Other multiple-ring positron cameras introduced recently include the four-detector-ring units manufactured by Scanditronix of Sweden and the three- and four-ring imaging systems offered by Cyclotron Corporation. A summary

Table 14-2.   *Some Commercially Available Positron Cameras*

Company	Model	Type	Crystal/Ring	No. of Rings	Slices
AECL[a]	3128	Head	64 BGO	2	3
Scanditronix[b]	PC 384	Head	96 BGO	4	7
	PC 512	Body	128 BGO	4	7
Cyclotron Corporation[c]	PC 4500	Body	128 BGO	4	7
	PC 4600	Head	96 BGO	5	9
	PC 4650	Head	96 BGO	3	5
EG&G-Ortec[d]	ECAT-II	Body	66 NaI	1 Hexagonal	1
	Neuro-ECAT	Head	88 BGO	3 Octagonal	5

[a]Atomic Energy of Canada Ltd., Medical Products, Ottawa, Canada.
[b]Scanditronix, Taby, Sweden; or Nucletronix, Gloucester, Mass.
[c]Cyclotron Corporation, Berkeley, Calif.
[d]EG&G-Ortec, Oak Ridge, Tenn.
Source: Reprinted from P. N. Goodwin, Recent developments in instrumentation for emission computed tomography. *Semin. Nucl. Med.* 10:322, 1980. With permission.

of some commercially available positron cameras is provided in Table 14-2. In addition, a positron tomographic unit for brain imaging (the Neuro-PET) has been developed by R. A. Brooks and co-workers [3] at the National Institutes of Health.

With newer scintillation detectors, which yield very short fluorescence decay times, the possibility has materialized for constructing positron cameras with *time-of-flight* capability. In this approach, differences are measured in the arrival times of annihilation photons at opposing detectors. From these measurements, the origin of the annihilation photons along a path between the two detectors can be determined [16]. A whole-body time-of-flight positron camera (PETT-VII) has been constructed at Washington University, and other investigators are exploring the concept. If the approach is successful, significant improvements may be possible in the spatial resolution of images obtained with positron tomographic units.

Cyclotrons

One of the major handicaps to positron imaging has been the need for a nearby cyclotron to produce the short-lived positron-emitting nuclides of interest in nuclear imaging. For example, the half-lives of ^{11}C, ^{13}N, and ^{15}O are 20, 10, and 2

Table 14-3. *Some Cyclotrons for In-Hospital Use*

| Manufacturer | Model | Particle Energies (MeV) | | Beam (μamp) |
		Protons	Deuterons	
Cyclotron Corp.[a]	CP-16	4–16	3–8	50,100
	CP-30	8–30	2–15	50,100
	CP-42	11–42	6–24	50,200
JSW/AECL[b]	10/7	10	7	50
	16/8	16	8	50
CGR MeV/SHI[c]	Cypris	13.6	8	10–50
Scanditronix[d]	MC 16F	16	8	50

[a]Cyclotron Corp., Berkeley, Calif.
[b]Atomic Energy of Canada Ltd., Medical Products, Ottawa, Canada.
[c]CGR MeV, Buc, France, or 2519 Wilkens Ave., Baltimore, Md.
[d]Scanditronix, Taby, Sweden; or Nucletronix, Gloucester, Mass.
Source: Reprinted from P. N. Goodwin, Recent developments in instrumentation for emission computed tomography. *Semin. Nucl. Med.* 10:322, 1980. With permission.

min respectively. Recently, several companies have developed compact cyclotrons, designed primarily for production of these positron emitters. Among companies marketing medical cyclotrons are the Cyclotron Corporation, Atomic Energy of Canada Ltd., Scanditronix (with its U.S. affiliate, Nucletronix), and CGR-France. The cost of a small cyclotron intended primarily for hospital use, including installation and a facility for radionuclide production, exceeds $1,000,000. Examples of cyclotrons for medical use are given in Table 14-3.

REFERENCES

1. Anger, H. O. The Scintillation Camera for Radioisotope Localization. In G. Hoffman and K. E. Sheer (eds.), *Radioisotope in der Lokalisations-Diagnostik*. Stuttgart: F. K. Schattauer-Verlag, 1967. P. 18.

2. Barrett, H. H. Fresnel zone plate imaging in nuclear medicine. *J. Nucl. Med.* 13:382, 1972.

3. Brooks, R. A., et al. Design of a high-resolution positron-emission tomograph: The Neuro-PET. *J. Comput. Assist. Tomogr.* 4:5, 1980.

4. Brownell, G. L., et al. Transverse Section Imaging of Radionuclide Distribution in Heart, Lung, and Brain. In M. M. Ter-Pogossian, et al. (eds.), *Reconstruction Tomography in Diagnostic Radiology and Nuclear Medicine*. Baltimore: University Park Press, 1977. P. 293.

5. Budinger, T. F. Quantitative Nuclear Medicine Imaging: Application of Computers to the Gamma Camera and Whole-Body Scanner. In J. Lawrence (ed.), *Recent Advances in Nuclear Medicine IV*. New York: Grune & Stratton, 1974. P. 41.

6. Budinger, T. F. and Gullberg, G. T. Transverse Section Reconstruction of Gamma-Ray–Emitting Radionuclides in Patients. In M. M. Ter-Pogossian, et al. (eds.), *Reconstruction Tomography in Diagnostic Radiology and Nuclear Medicine*. Baltimore: University Park Press, 1977. P. 315.

7. Budinger, T. F. Physical attributes of single-photon tomography. *J. Nucl. Med.* 21:579, 1980.

8. Carroll, L. R. Design and performance characteristics of a production model positron imaging system. *IEEE Nucl. Sci.* NS-25:606, 1978.

9. Chang, W., Lin, S. L., and Henkin, R. E. A Rotatable Quadrant Slant-Hole Collimator for Tomography (QSH): A Stationary Scintillation Camera Based Spect System. *Single-Photon Emission Computed Tomography and Other Selected Computer Topics*. New York: Society of Nuclear Medicine, 1980. P. 81.

10. Chang, W., Lin, S. L., and Henkin, R. E. A Comparison of the Performance Parameters of the Seven-Pinhole Collimator and the Quadrant Slant-Hole Collimator (QSH). *Single-Photon Emission Computed Tomography and Other Selected Computer Topics*. New York: Society of Nuclear Medicine, 1980. P. 113.

11. Freedman, G. S. Gamma camera tomography. Theory and preliminary clinical experience. *Radiology* 102:365, 1972.

12. Goodwin, P. N. Recent developments in instrumentation for emission computed tomography. *Semin. Nucl. Med.* 10:322, 1980.

13. Hendee, W. R. *Medical Radiation Physics* (2nd ed.). Chicago: Year Book, 1979. P. 287.

14. Hill, T. C., et al. Early clinical experience with a radionuclide emission computed tomographic brain-imaging system. *Radiology* 128:803, 1978.

15. Hoffman, E. J., Huang, S-C., and Phelps, M. E. Quantitation in positron-emission computed tomography. I. Effect of object size. *J. Comput. Assist. Tomogr.* 3:299, 1979.

16. Joseph, P. M., and Spital, R. D. A method for correcting bone-induced artifacts in computed tomography scanners. *J. Comput. Assist. Tomogr.* 2:100, 1978.

162

17. Kan, M. K., and Hopkins, G. B. Measurement of liver volume by emission computed tomography. *J. Nucl. Med.* 20:514, 1979.

18. Kay, D. B., Keyes, J. W., Jr., and Simon, W. Radionuclide tomographic image reconstruction using Fourier transform techniques. *J. Nucl. Med.* 15:981, 1974.

19. Keyes, J. W., Jr., et al. Myocardial infarct quantification in the dog by single-photon emission computed tomography. *Circulation* 58:227, 1978.

20. Keyes, J. W., Jr., et al. The "Humongotron"—a scintillation-camera transaxial tomograph. *J. Nucl. Med.* 18:381, 1977.

21. Kuhl, D. E., and Edwards, R. Q. Image separation radioisotope scanning. *Radiology* 80:653, 1963.

22. Kuhl, D. E., et al. Quantitative section scanning using orthogonal tangent correction. *J. Nucl. Med.* 14:196, 1973.

23. Muehllehner, G. A tomographic scintillation camera. *Phys. Med. Biol.* 16:87, 1971.

24. Mullani, N. A., Ficke, D. C., and Ter-Pogossian, M. M. Cesium fluoride: A new detector for positron-emission tomography. *IEEE Nucl. Sci.* NS-27:572, 1980.

25. Murphy, P. H., et al. Radionuclide computed tomography of the body using routine radiopharmaceuticals. I. System Characterization. *J. Nucl. Med.* 20:102, 1979.

26. Oppenheim, B. E. More accurate algorithms for iterative three-dimensional reconstruction. *IEEE Trans. Nucl. Sci.* NS-21:72, 1974.

27. Rogers, W. L., et al. Coded-aperture imaging of the heart. *J. Nucl. Med.* 21:371, 1980.

28. Ter-Pogossian, M. M., Raichle, M. E., and Sobel, B. E. Positron-emission tomography. *Sci. Am.* 243:170, 1980 (Oct.).

29. Vogel, R. A., et al. A new method of multiplanar emission tomography using a seven-pinhole collimator and an Anger scintillation camera. *J. Nucl. Med.* 19:648, 1978.

30. Weiss, E. S., et al. Quantification of infarction in cross sections of canine myocardium in vivo with positron-emission transaxial tomography and ^{11}C-palmitate. *Circulation* 55:66, 1977.

15

Computed Tomography with Ultrasound

Ultrasonic computed tomography (CT) is being investigated as a potential imaging method for certain tissues in the body that are accessible to transmitted ultrasound. Among these tissues are the female breast, the male genitals, the infant head, and, possibly, certain parts of the extremities such as the wrist. The clinical utility of ultrasonic (CT) remains to be determined, although the results to date appear promising.

PRINCIPLES OF ULTRASONIC CT

Ultrasonic CT uses pulses of ultrasound energy transmitted through the body part to be imaged, in much the same way as transmitted x rays are used to form transaxial images in x-ray computed tomography. Work to date with ultrasonic CT has used pencil-like and fan-shaped ultrasound beams and a simple translate-rotate geometry for data acquisition similar to that employed in first-generation x-ray CT scanners. Although more sophisticated geometries, such as purely rotational motion, have not been attempted, there is no reason to believe that they are not adaptable to ultrasonic CT imaging.

An ultrasonic CT scanner is depicted in Figure 15-1. Two ultrasound transducers are suspended in a water-filled phantom, with one transducer serving as a transmitter of ultrasound energy, and the second receiving the transmitted energy. The transducers usually are relatively large in diameter and are moderately focused to yield reasonable spatial resolution at the depths of interest in the patient and efficient collection of ultrasound energy by the receiving transducer. The body part to be imaged is suspended from above between the two transducers, and the transducers scan in synchrony from one side of the body part to the other. Typically, 100 pulses of transmitted ultrasound are measured during a single translation of the transmitting and receiving transducers. The angular

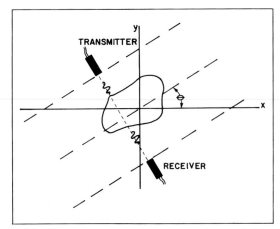

FIGURE 15-1. *Representation of an ultrasound CT scanner.*

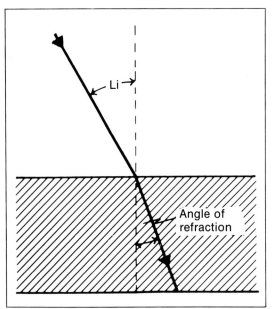

FIGURE 15-2. *Illustration of refraction of an ultrasound beam at an interface between different media. (Reproduced with permission from W. R. Hendee, Ultrasound Waves.* Medical Radiation Physics: Roentgenology, Nuclear Medicine, and Ultrasound [2nd ed.]. *Chicago: Year Book, 1979. Chap. 20, p. 401. Copyright © 1979 by Year Book Medical Publishers, Inc., Chicago.)*

orientation of the transducers is then changed slightly (e.g., 2 degrees), and a second translational scan is obtained. This scanning process is repeated at additional angular increments through 180 degrees, resulting in approximately 9,000 measurements of transmitted ultrasound. From these measurements, a tomographic image is reconstructed in the manner employed in x-ray CT. In most cases, the reconstruction algorithm is modeled from the convolution technique developed by G. N. Ramachandran and A. V. Laksminarayanan [14] and described earlier in Chapter 5.

A number of ultrasonic characteristics of tissues may be measured by transmission CT with ultrasound. For example, some studies of ultrasonic CT have produced attenuation images similar to those obtained in x-ray CT [4]. For these studies, transmission data are obtained by measuring the amplitude of ultrasound pulses traversing the body part and impinging on the receiving transducer. From these transmission data, attenuation images are reconstructed that are displayed either as numerical attenuation data or as gray-scale images. However, the images are distorted rather severely by refraction of the ultrasound beam at interfaces between tissues with different speeds of sound. The bending, or refraction, of an ultrasound beam at an interface is described by Snell's law; refraction is depicted in Figure 15-2.

Snell's law is expressed as follows:

$$\frac{\text{Angle of incidence}}{\text{Angle of refraction}} = \frac{\text{Velocity in incident medium}}{\text{Velocity in refractive medium}}$$

In spite of the problems inherent in attenuation imaging with ultrasound, the clinical usefulness of ultrasonic attenuation images continues to be of interest, and investigators are exploring methods to reduce the image artifacts and degradation caused by refraction and reflection. In spite of these efforts, refraction and reflection are

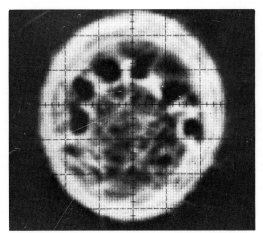

FIGURE 15-3.   *Ultrasonic transaxial tomographic image of the attenuation of ultrasound in the female breast. (Courtesy of P. L. Carson and A. L. Scherzinger.)*

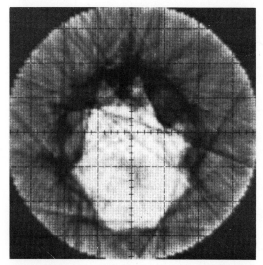

FIGURE 15-4.   *Speed of sound image of the same tomographic plane and patient as the attenuation image depicted in Figure 15-3. (Courtesy of P. L. Carson and A. L. Scherzinger.)*

the major limitations in the spatial resolution of attenuation images with transmitted ultrasound. An ultrasound attenuation image of the female breast is shown in Figure 15-3.

Compared to ultrasonic attenuation, a somewhat more promising ultrasound characteristic for clinical purposes is the speed of ultrasound through different tissues comprising a particular body part. This characteristic is determined by measuring the transit time of the leading edge of an ultrasound pulse through the body part. Transit time measurements are obtained at different translational positions and angular orientations, and a matrix of ultrasound speeds is computed by a reconstruction process identical to that used for attenuation reconstruction. Speed-of-sound reconstructions have been compiled by J. F. Greenleaf and co-workers at the Mayo Clinic [5], by G. H. Glover and J. C. Sharp at General Electric [3], and by P. L. Carson and colleagues at the Universities of Colorado and Michigan [1]. A speed-of-sound tomographic image of the female breast is shown in Figure 15-4.

An advantage of ultrasound CT is that a variety of ultrasonic characteristics of tissue can be measured simultaneously. Shown in Figure 15-5 are B-mode reflection, attenuation CT and speed-of-sound CT images obtained simultaneously through the same tomographic section of the female breast. Since each of these images depicts different ultrasonic characteristics of tissue, their simultaneous acquisition may be more useful clinically than any single characteristic measured separately.

In addition to attenuation and ultrasonic speed, other ultrasonic characteristics of tissue have been proposed for ultrasound CT reconstruction techniques. Among these characteristics are changes in ultrasonic attenuation with changing frequency of the ultrasonic pulse [11]; absorption of ultrasound, as distinguished from attenuation of ultrasound, in biologic tissues; and acoustic impedance. Reconstruction tech-

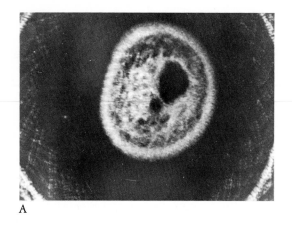

A

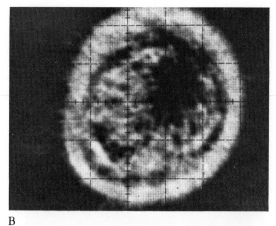

B

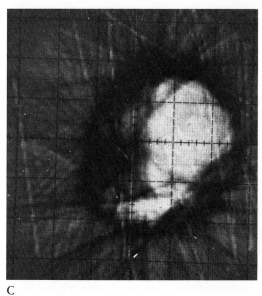

C

FIGURE 15-5. *B-mode reflection (a), attenuation CT (b), and speed-of-sound CT images (c) obtained simultaneously through a tomographic section of the female breast. (Courtesy of P. L. Carson and A. L. Scherzinger.)*

niques also have been proposed for quantitative determination of ultrasound scattering [2] and for measurement of the velocity of moving fluids in the body. From time-of-flight measurements, it may be possible to obtain tomographic maps of the temperature distribution in tissues [8] and to determine corrections for ultrasound refraction in B-mode reflection and CT attenuation images [6, 12]. Determination of these characteristics and corrections will require techniques for analysis of transmitted ultrasonic signals that are considerably more sophisticated than those used for simple attenuation and speed-of-sound reconstruction. These techniques may not materialize until considerably more information becomes available concerning the fundamental interactions of ultrasonic energy in biologic tissue. Initial applications of more sophisticated techniques for signal analysis include iterative corrections for refraction of the ultrasound beam [8] and reconstruction algorithms that assume weak scattering of the beam [12]. Other efforts to characterize ultrasonic properties of tissues by reconstruction techniques include the work of S. M. Jones and co-workers [9], and A. C. Kak and K. A. Dines [10].

Since bone and gas interfere with ultrasound transmission, CT employing transmitted beams of ultrasound energy probably is limited to anatomic sites where these disturbing influences are not present. Among these sites are the female breast, the male genitals, and the infant head. Application of ultrasonic CT to other body parts probably requires the development of reconstruction methods utilizing reflected, rather than transmitted, ultrasound. Preliminary exploration of this possibility is underway; however, reflection reconstruction techniques are considerably more complicated than those employing transmitted ultrasound [2, 13]. To date, ultrasound computed tomography has focused primarily on transmission reconstruction images of the breast. Although the clinical usefulness of this application remains to be determined, initial results are promising, especially in combination with B-mode reflection images [1, 7].

REFERENCES

1. Carson, P. L., et al. Progress in ultrasonic computed tomography (CT) of the breast. *Application of Optical Instrumentation in Medicine VII*, Vol. 173. Bellingham, Wash.: Society of Photo-Optical Engineers, 1979. P. 372.

2. Duck, F. A., and Hill, C. R. Mapping True Ultrasonic Backscatter and Attenuation Distributions in Tissue. A Digital Reconstruction Approach. In M. Linzer (ed.), *Ultrasonic Tissue Characterization II*, NBS Spec. Pub. 525. Washington, D.C.: U.S. Govt. Printing Office, 1979. P. 247.

3. Glover, G. H., and Sharp, J. C. Reconstruction of ultrasound propagation speed distributions in soft tissue: Time-of-flight tomography. *IEEE Trans. Sonics and Ultrasonics* 24:229, 1977.

4. Greenleaf, J. F., et al. Algebraic Reconstruction of Spatial Distributions of Acoustic Absorption Within Tissue from Their Two-Dimensional Acoustic Projections. In P. S. Green (ed.), *Acoustical Holography*. New York: Plenum Press, 1975. Vol. 5, P. 541.

5. Greenleaf, J. F., et al. Algebraic reconstruction of spatial distributions of acoustic velocities in tissue from their time-of-flight profiles. In P. S. Green (ed.), *Acoustical Holography*. New York: Plenum Press, 1974. Vol. 5, P. 71.

6. Greenleaf, J. F., et al. Refractive Index by Reconstruction: Use to Improve Compound B-scan Resolution. In P. S. Green (ed.), *Acoustical Holography*. New York: Plenum Press, 1977. Vol. 7, P. 263.

7. Greenleaf, J. F., and Bahn, R. C. Clinical imaging with transmissive ultrasonic computerized tomography. *IEEE Trans. Biomed. Engr.* BME-28, 1981.

8. Johnson, S. A., et al. Reconstruction of Three-Dimensional Velocity Fields and Other Parameters by Acoustic Ray Tracing. *IEEE Ultrasound Symp. Proc.* (IEEE No. 75, CH0994-7SU), 1975. P. 46.

9. Jones, S. M., et al. Investigation of Phase-Incoherent and Other Signal Processing with a Simulated Array for Ultrasonic CT. Proc. IEEE-EMBS Conf. Frontiers of Engineering in Health Care, Oct. 1979.

10. Kak, A. C., and Dines, K. A. Signal processing of broad-band pulsed ultrasound: Measurement of attenuation of soft biological tissues. *IEEE Trans. Biomed. Engr.* 25:321, 1978.

11. Klepper, J. K., et al. Phase-Cancellation, Reflection, and Refraction Effects in Quantitative Ultrasonic Attenuation Tomography. Proc. IEEE Ultrasound Symp. (IEEE No. 77, CH1264-1SU), 182, 1977.

12. Mueller, R. K., Kaveh, M., and Wade, G. Acoustical reconstruction tomography. *IEEE Proc.* 67:567, 1979.

13. Norton, S. J., and Linzer, M. Tomographic reconstruction of reflectivity images (abstract). 3rd International Symp. on Ultrasound Imaging and Tissue Characterization. Gaithersburg, Maryland, June 5–6, 1978.

14. Ramachandran, G. N., and Laksminarayanan, A. V. Three-dimensional reconstruction from radiographs and electron micrographs: Application of convolution instead of Fourier transforms. *Proc. Natl. Acad. Sci.* 68:2236, 1971.

16

Nuclear Magnetic-Resonance Imaging

Since the mid-1940s, nuclear magnetic resonance (NMR) has been used by physicists and chemists to analyze the structure of complex chemical configurations such as organic and biochemical molecules. For the development of NMR, F. Bloch and E. M. Purcell were awarded the Nobel Prize in physics in 1952 [5, 25]. More recently, NMR techniques have been used to study the biochemistry of living tissues. For example, NMR helps to characterize the metabolic activity of tissues by identifying changes in the concentration of phosphate compounds in the tissues. This identification promises to characterize alterations in the enzymatic activity of tissues that reflect disease processes and their treatment by drugs [8, 23]. Even in vivo analyses of certain aspects of the biochemistry of internal organs appear to be attainable. For example, McArdle's syndrome, a rare genetic condition accompanied by changes in the phosphate biochemistry of skeletal muscle, appears to be susceptible to diagnosis by NMR [26]. Of even greater significance is the potential of NMR to depict the extent of damage in heart-attack and stroke victims and the response of these patients to physical and drug therapy.

None of the NMR applications described above involves the formation of images. The potential of NMR as an imaging modality was not recognized until P. C. Lauterbur's 1973 paper [21] on the subject, although the promise of NMR as a method for cancer detection had been speculated on by R. Damadian two years earlier [11]. Since 1973, extensive effort has been directed toward development of NMR as an imaging modality, and today NMR images are comparable to those provided by x-ray transmission computed tomography. The diagnostic usefulness of these images, however, remains to be documented.

Imaging with NMR is a complex technology

that is strongly dependent on magnet and computer technology. Consequently, considerable capital investment is needed to equip a clinical facility for NMR imaging, on the order of at least that required for x-ray computed tomography. In addition, to realize the full potential of this promising development in medical imaging, skilled technologists and a labor-intensive interaction of physicists, technologists, and physicians is required.

PRINCIPLES OF NMR

All nuclei possess the properties of *positive charge* and *spin*. In nuclei with odd numbers of protons or neutrons, these properties produce a *net* (composite) *magnetic moment* much like that exhibited by a small magnet. When many nuclei are present in a sample, their magnetic moments are oriented randomly, so no composite magnetic moment exists for the sample (Figure 16-1A). When the sample is placed in an external magnetic field, however, a composite magnetic moment is produced because the nuclei tend to line up more or less parallel to the field as if they were small magnets (Figure 16-1B). By applying a second radiofrequency-alternating magnetic field to the samples, the composite magnetic moment of the aligned nuclei can be "flipped" out of alignment with the external field (Figure 16-1C). This flipped magnetic moment precesses around the direction of the applied field, much as a top precesses around its axis of rotation, especially when it is slowing down (Figure 16-1D). The frequency of the precessional motion is termed the *Larmor precessional frequency*. The Larmor frequency ν varies with the intensity B of the magnetic field at the location of the nuclei according to the relationship $\nu = \gamma B$, where γ is a constant known as the *gyromagnetic* (or magnetogyric) *ratio of the nuclei*.

Once the precessional motion of the composite magnetic moment has begun, a small (a few nanovolts) electrical signal can be detected by

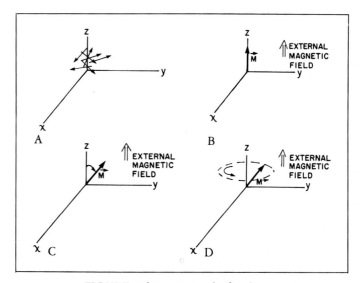

FIGURE 16-1.   *Principle of nuclear magnetic reso-*
nance. A. Sample with randomly oriented magnetic mo-
ments. B. Alignment of the net magnetic moment of the
sample in an external magnetic field. C. Flipping of the
net magnetic moment from its equilibrium position by im-
position of an rf magnetic field. D. Precession of the net
magnetic moment around the direction of the applied field.

placing a coil around the sample. This signal decreases over time with a characteristic time constant (Figure 16-2) termed the *spin-spin relaxation time* T_2 of the sample. The decay of the signal is caused by interactions among nuclei with flipped magnetic moments that cause a dephasing of the assembly of nuclei (Figure 16-3A). In addition, the composite magnetic moment also realigns rather rapidly with the applied magnetic field (Figure 16-3B). The time constant T_1 that describes this realignment is known as the *spin-lattice relaxation time* T_1. The relaxation time T_1 is a reflection of the interaction between nuclei with flipped magnetic moments and the environment or "lattice" of the nuclei. In all samples, $T_1 \geqslant T_2$, with the time constants exhibiting greater differences in solids than in liquids. In ice, for example, T_1 is measured in minutes and T_2 is measured in microseconds, whereas in water both time constants are on the order of a few seconds [6].

The electrical signal induced in a pickup coil by the precessing magnetic moment has a characteristic frequency equal to the Larmor precessional frequency. This frequency (or frequencies for a chemically complex sample) can be plotted as a frequency spectrum as shown in Figure 16-4. The width $\Delta \nu$ of the frequency peak at half of its maximum amplitude is a measure of T_2 according to the relationship $\Delta \nu = 2/T_2$, and the frequency at the maximum amplitude of the peak is the Larmor precessional frequency. The area under the frequency peak reflects the intensity of the magnetic field at the location of the sample and the concentration of nuclei in the sample.

The Larmor precessional frequency depends on the local magnetic field and, hence, on such local conditions as molecular structure, pH, temperature, and other variables. An NMR frequency spectrum for muscle is shown in Figure 16-5 as an example. In this spectrum, separate peaks are shown for the phosphorus-containing compounds adenosine triphosphate (ATP),

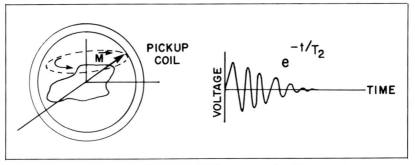

FIGURE 16-2.   *A sample with a precessing magnetic moment induces an alternating voltage in pickup coils placed around the sample (left). The voltage oscillates with the Larmor precessional frequency and decays with characteristic time constants T_1 and T_2 (right).*

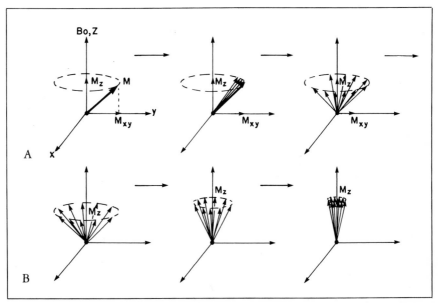

FIGURE 16-3.   *Loss of the flipped alignment of the sample magnetic moment with respect to the external magnetic field. A. Dephasing of the nuclear magnetic moments characterized by the time constant T_2. B. Realignment of the nuclear magnetic moments characterized by the time constant T_1. (Reproduced from D. I. Hoult,* An Overview of NMR in Medicine. *NCHCT Monograph, U.S. Dept. Health and Human Services, Washington, D.C., 1981. With permission.)*

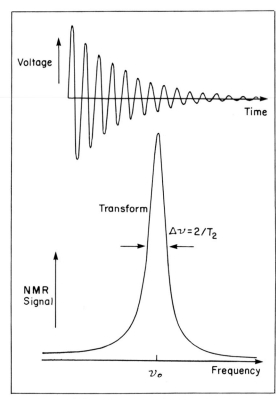

FIGURE 16-4. *Frequency spectrum for a typical NMR signal. The spin-spin relaxation time T_2, the Larmor precessional frequency v, and the concentration of an element of interest in the sample can be determined from this spectrum. (Reproduced from D. I. Hoult,* An Overview of NMR in Medicine. NCHCT *Monograph, U.S. Dept. Health and Human Services, Washington, D.C., 1981. With permission.)*

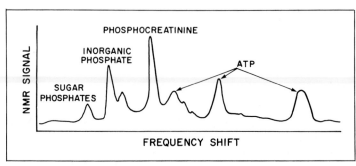

FIGURE 16-5. *Representative NMR frequency spectrum for skeletal muscle.*

Table 16-1. *NMR Sensitivity to Various Isotopes in Biologic Tissues Relative to Hydrogen*

Isotope	NMR Sensitivity
^1H	1.000
^2H	6.2×10^{-5}
B	7.3×10^{-7}
C	2.5×10^{-4}
^{14}N	3.1×10^{-3}
^{15}N	6.0×10^{-6}
O	4.9×10^{-4}
F	6.3×10^{-5}
Na	10^{-3}
Mg	7×10^{-6}
Al	9×10^{-7}
Si	9.2×10^{-8}
P	1.4×10^{-3}
S	1.1×10^{-6}
Cl	8.4×10^{-5}
K	1.1×10^{-4}
Ca	9.1×10^{-6}
Fe	5.2×10^{-9}
Cu	8.5×10^{-8}
Zn	1.8×10^{-7}
Rb	4.3×10^{-7}
Sr	2.6×10^{-7}
I	2.0×10^{-8}
Ba	2.6×10^{-9}
Pb	3×10^{-9}

Source: Adapted with permission from D. M. Kramer, Imaging of Elements Other than Hydrogen. In L. Kaufman, L. W. Crooks, and A. R. Margulis (eds.), *Nuclear Magnetic Resonance Imaging in Medicine.* Tokyo: Igaku-Shoin, 1981. P. 184.

phosphocreatine, inorganic phosphate, and sugar phosphates.

In biologic tissue, the strongest NMR signal is produced by hydrogen, primarily because this element is so plentiful in organic molecules and because the NMR signal is inherently larger for hydrogen than for other elements. The sensitivity of NMR to other elements in biologic tissues is described in Table 16-1, with hydrogen assigned a relative value of 1. In this table, the NMR sensitivity is the product of the average molar concentration of the element in tissue, the natural abundance of the element's isotope that yields an NMR signal, and the intrinsic relative sensitivity of the isotope to magnetic-field influences imposed during the NMR process. Exceptions to the average molar concentration may exist for certain tissues and organs that concentrate specific elements.

The use of NMR to detect elements other than hydrogen is primarily a problem of separating the desired signals from background noise. To accomplish this separation, static magnetic fields are required that are more intense than those used to detect hydrogen. For example, the detection of phosphorus requires a magnetic-field intensity at least 2.5 times that used for hydrogen, whereas the detection of sodium or carbon requires an increase of about ×4 in magnetic field intensity. To apply these stronger magnetic fields uniformly over large volumes of tissue, superconducting magnets are required. Superconducting magnets are expensive to build and operate. In addition, sudden collapse of the magnetic field caused by a loss of power in a superconducting magnet could create a hazard to the patient [7].

ELEMENTS SUSCEPTIBLE TO NMR IMAGING

Hydrogen in the body occurs to the greatest extent in body water, and NMR images of hydrogen depict primarily the distribution of this tissue constituent. To a lesser degree, NMR images of hydrogen portray the lipid content of tissues. Excluding hydrogen, the most promising elements for NMR imaging are nitrogen, phosphorus, sodium, oxygen, carbon, potassium, chlorine, and fluorine [9, 18].

Nitrogen (^{14}N and ^{15}N) is one of the commoner elements in biologic tissues and might be considered as a reasonable candidate for NMR imaging. However, most nitrogen is present as ^{14}N, and this isotope yields an NMR signal with a wide range of frequencies, especially when it is incorporated into complex molecules.

Consequently, it is difficult to isolate nitrogen signals from background noise and from signals from other elements, and the prospects for NMR imaging of nitrogen appear rather poor. Although the range of signal frequencies is somewhat narrower for nitrogen incorporated into lighter compounds such as amino acids or urea, the concentration of these substances in the body is very low, and the resulting NMR signals also are difficult to separate from background noise.

Phosphorus (^{31}P) is probably the most promising element for NMR imaging after hydrogen. This element yields NMR signals with a narrow range of frequencies and offers the opportunity to distinguish phosphorus-containing compounds such as ADP and ATP, phosphocreatinine, sugar phosphates, and inorganic phosphate. Because of the low NMR sensitivity to these chemical forms of phosphorus, signal-to-noise ratios are low, and phosphorus images undoubtedly will exhibit poor image quality. Nevertheless, studies are underway to determine the clinical utility of phosphorus NMR measurements as a diagnostic tool and possibly as an imaging modality [24].

Sodium (^{23}Na) yields an NMR sensitivity of about one-thousandth that of hydrogen. Nevertheless, this element may be susceptible to NMR imaging, because the concentration of sodium varies widely from one biologic tissue to another. For example, the concentration of sodium in brain is more than twice that in muscle, the kidneys contain less than one-fifth of the sodium in muscle, and the concentration of sodium is 25 percent greater in liver than in muscle. Because of these wide variations in sodium concentration, a lower signal-to-noise ratio can be tolerated for NMR imaging of sodium.

Oxygen (^{17}O), *Potassium* (^{39}K), and *Chlorine* (^{35}Cl) are similar to sodium in their potential for NMR imaging, except that the signals will be even weaker. Compared to sodium, the tissue concentrations of potassium and chlorine are lower, and the NMR sensitivity is reduced. The signals from oxygen are weak because the natural abundance of ^{17}O is low. Although these elements have been considered for NMR studies of proteins and solutions, their potential for imaging appears limited. Signals from oxygen primarily reflect the body distribution of water, and this substance is characterized much better by NMR imaging of hydrogen.

Carbon (^{13}C) is not a very promising isotope for NMR imaging because the signals from even a rather simple hydrocarbon are complex and difficult to interpret. Although diets containing ^{13}C-enriched nutrients have been proposed as a way to enhance the NMR analysis of carbon, the high cost of these nutrients prohibits their widespread use.

Fluorine (^{19}F) yields an NMR signal that encompasses a wide range of frequencies. For this reason, and because fluorine is present almost exclusively in teeth and bone and is virtually absent in soft tissue, little attention has been paid to the prospect of NMR imaging of this element. However, the absence of fluorine in soft tissue suggests that a fluorine-containing compound, such as a fluorocarbon introduced as a tracer into soft tissue or the cardiovascular system, might yield useful information since it could be detected in the virtual absence of noise [15].

In general, NMR imaging of elements other than hydrogen is subject to serious technical difficulties as well as uncertain clinical usefulness. Exceptions to this generalization may exist for sodium, phosphorus, and, possibly, fluorine. Because of low signal-to-noise ratios, the resolution of NMR images of elements such as potassium, chlorine, nitrogen, and oxygen is limited to a few centimeters and probably does not justify much exploration. Although the use of NMR to image sodium and phosphorus is somewhat more promising, intense and more uniform magnetic fields will be required for these images. In addition, signal-to-noise ratios will be much lower for these elements than for hydrogen, and the quality of the images will be poor.

CHARACTERISTICS OF IN VIVO NMR MEASUREMENTS

Three parameters of biologic tissues that can be reflected in NMR images are the density of hydrogen atoms (or other elemental constituents) in the tissues, and the relaxation times T_1 and T_2. The relaxation times describe the equilibration of nuclei of the element of interest (e.g., hydrogen) with other nuclei (T_2), and with the overall environment of the sample (T_1).

The values of T_1 and T_2 differ for various tissues, depending on the physical and chemical environment of the element under investigation. By analysis of these differences, the concentration of the element in one tissue can be differentiated from that in other tissues. For example, hydrogen in blood can be distinguished from hydrogen in tissues such as muscle; hence NMR may be useful for measurement of myocardial and brain perfusion [10]. Other applications of this approach might include the use of NMR to delineate fluid-filled cysts and pulmonary edema, and to differentiate blood from extracellular and intracellular fluids. The latter application might be helpful in identifying lesions that differ from normal tissue in blood perfusion or extracellular fluid space [9].

In 1971, Damadian [11] suggested that spin-lattice relaxation times T_1 are longer in tumors than in normal tissues. This suggestion has produced considerable speculation concerning the application of NMR to cancer detection. In some cases, NMR measurements in vitro do reveal differences between cancerous tissue and normal tissue extracted from an adjacent region. However, it is doubtful that cancerous tissue can be identified solely from T_1 values measured in vivo without comparison to T_1 measurements for normal tissues from the same person, since biologic and technique variability are uncontrolled under these circumstances.

Because T_1 and T_2 values for hydrogen are related to the freedom of motion of water molecules, it has been suggested that the concentration of structurally bound water is different in cancerous, as compared to normal, tissues. This difference in bound water has even been postulated to extend to noncancerous organs and to the sera of tumor-bearing animals and humans. This whole-body response to cancer, termed a *systemic effect* [4], might lead to elevated T_1 values for the sera of cancer patients, and might serve as a mechanism for cancer detection. Investigators of this possibility have concluded, however, that elevation of serum T_1 values probably reflects a variety of disease states and is not a specific indication of cancer [16].

NMR is used widely in industry to measure flow rates, and it has been applied with limited success to the measurement of blood flow in humans [2, 3]. The technique involves "tagging" a bolus of blood in vivo by inverting its magnetization with a small coil placed over a vessel. Detection of this bolus of tagged blood with a second coil positioned downstream along the vessel provides an estimate of the flow rate of blood through the vessel. The method is limited by low sensitivity and by the limited time before the state of inverted magnetization disappears.

NMR imaging is currently the most widely discussed application of NMR to medicine. This mode of imaging is sometimes referred to as *NUMAR* or *zeugmatography* (derived from the Greek for "that which joins together"). The principle of NMR imaging is implicit in the relationship between the strength of the external magnetic field B and the Larmor precessional frequency ν: $\nu = \gamma B$.

When a individual is placed in a magnetic field with a gradient of increasing field strength, signals of higher frequency are detected at the

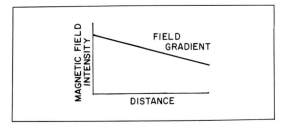

FIGURE 16-6.   *For NMR imaging, a gradient in magnetic field intensity is required across the sample. The frequency of the voltage induced in the pickup coils varies with the intensity of the magnetic field as the coils are scanned across the sample in the direction of the gradient.*

more intense end of the applied field, and lower frequency signals are detected at the opposite end (Figure 16-6). If more intense signals are received at the higher-frequency end of the applied field, a higher concentration of hydrogen (or other element of interest) must be present at that end. With this technique, a one-dimensional map of elemental concentration versus distance can be obtained. By repeating the process with the magnetic-field gradient oriented in different directions, sets of elemental concentration data can be obtained. These sets of data can then be combined by computed tomographic techniques to furnish a two- or three-dimensional image of the distribution of the element in the patient. For example, if the element of interest is hydrogen, the image reveals the distribution of water (and, to a lesser extent, of fat) in the person.

Four distinct approaches have been developed to accumulate the data needed for NMR images. The first, developed by R. Damadian [12] and W. S. Hinshaw [14], utilizes a small sample volume that is scanned through the patient to provide the data required for reconstruction. This method, referred to as the *sensitive-point technique*, is simple but requires scanning times of 10 min or so to accumulate the data for a single planar image. The second approach, involving the simultaneous accumulation of one or more lines of data, was pioneered by E. R. Andrew [1] and P. Mansfield [22] and their colleagues. The method provides faster scan times than the sensitive-point method. The third method permits simultaneous accumulation of NMR data from an entire plane. This method is more efficient than the other two approaches, but it is more difficult to implement. Developers of this approach include R. C. Hawkes and co-workers [13]; A. Kumar, D. Welti, and R. R. Ernst [19]; and D. I. Hoult [17]. Images in Figure 16-7 were obtained with the planar method of data acquisition. The fourth approach involves the collection of data simultaneously

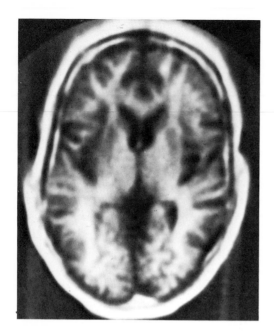 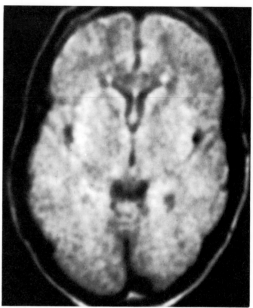

FIGURE 16-7. *NMR head images obtained at Hammersmith Hospital in London. (Courtesy of Picker International.)*

from an entire sample. This is the most complex approach of all; and it is being pursued only by C-M. Lai and P. C. Lauterbur [20] at the present time.

The spatial resolution of NMR images is influenced by a number of factors. These include the accuracy with which the Larmor frequency can be related to the gradient of the external magnetic field and the spatial precision of collecting NMR signals from the anatomic area of interest. Moreover, the relaxation times T_1 and T_2 and the overall signal-to-noise ratio of the NMR signals affect the spatial resolution, as does the amount of patient motion occurring while data are being accumulated for an NMR image. In spite of these influences, spatial resolution as fine as 1 to 2 mm may be achievable in 5-mm-thick sections for scanning times of less than 1 min [16]. To obtain three-dimensional information, much longer scanning times will probably be required. One of the intriguing possibilities of NMR is its promise to combine images with localized measurements of elemental concentrations and relaxation times to provide biochemical and metabolic, as well as anatomic, information.

POSSIBLE BIOEFFECTS OF NMR

Considerable effort currently is focused on identification of possible bioeffects associated with the magnetic fields used in NMR imaging. Three characteristics of the magnetic fields must be considered: the static field, the radiofrequency alternating magnetic field, and the gradient of the static field [7]. To date, no adverse physiologic effects have been noted at the intensities, frequencies, and gradients employed in NMR imaging. Of special concern are possible effects induced by sudden collapse of the magnetic field during a power failure, and the influence of metal devices such as prostheses that may be present in the patient.

REFERENCES

1. Andrew, E. R., et al. NMR images by the multiple sensitive-point method: Application to larger biological systems. *Phys. Med. Biol.* 22:971, 1977.

2. Battocletti, J. H., et al. Clinical applications and theoretical analysis of NMR blood flowmeter. *Biomed. Eng.* January, 1975.

3. Battocletti, J. H., et al. Flat crossed-coil detector for blood-flow measurement using nuclear magnetic resonance. *Med. Biol. Eng. Comput.* 17:183, 1979.

4. Beall, P. T., et al. Systemic effect of benign and malignant mammary tumors on the spin-lattice relaxation time of water protons in mouse serum. *J. Natl. Cancer Inst.* 59:1431, 1977.

5. Bloch, F. The principle of nuclear induction. *Science* 118:425, 1953.

6. Brown, P. W. NMR: Out of R & D and into radiology. *Diag. Imaging* 3:32, 1981.

7. Budinger, T. F. Nuclear magnetic resonance (NMR) thresholds for physiological effects due to rf and magnetic fields used in NMR imaging. *IEEE Trans. Nucl. Sci.* NS-26:2821, 1979.

8. Burt, C. T., Glonek, T., and Bárány, M. Analysis of living tissue by phosphorus-31 magnetic resonance. *Science* 195:145, 1977.

9. Crooks, L., et al. Tomography of hydrogen with NMR and the potential for imaging other body constituents. *SPIE Proc.* 206:120, 1979.

10. Crooks, L., and Singer, J. R. Some magnetic studies of normal and leukemic blood. *J. Clin. Eng.* 3:237, 1978.

11. Damadian, R. Tumor detection by nuclear magnetic resonance. *Science* 171:1151, 1971.

12. Damadian, R., et al. Field focusing nuclear magnetic resonance (FONAR): Visualization of a tumor in a live animal. *Science* 194:1430, 1976.

13. Hawkes, R. C., et al. Nuclear magnetic resonance (NMR) tomography of the brain: A preliminary clinical assessment with demonstration of pathology. *J. Comput. Assist. Tomogr.* 4:577, 1980.

14. Hinshaw, W. S. Spin mapping—the application of moving gradients to NMR. *Phys. Letters* 48A:87, 1974.

15. Holland, G. N., Bottomley, P. A., and Hinshaw, W. S. ^{19}F magnetic resonance imaging. *J. Magn. Res.* 28:133, 1977.

16. Hoult, D. I. An overview of NMR in medicine. NCHCT Monograph. Washington, D.C.: U.S. Dept. Health and Human Services, 1981.

17. Hoult, D. I. Rotating frame zeugmatography. *J. Magn. Res.* 33:183, 1979.

18. Kramer, D. M. Imaging of Elements Other Than Hydrogen. In L. Kaufman, L. W. Crooks, and A. R. Margulis (eds.), *Nuclear Magnetic Resonance Imaging in Medicine*. Tokyo: Igaku-Shoin, 1981. P. 184.

19. Kumar, A., Welti, D., and Ernst, R. R. NMR-Fourier zeugmatography. *J. Magn. Res.* 18:69, 1975.

20. Lai, C-M., and Lauterbur, P. C. True three-dimensional image reconstruction by nuclear magnetic resonance zeugmatography. *Phys. Med. Biol.* 26:851, 1981.

21. Lauterbur, P. C. Image formation by induced local interactions: Examples employing nuclear magnetic resonance. *Nature* 242:190, 1973.

22. Mansfield, P., and Pykett, I. L. Biological and medical imaging by NMR. *J. Magn. Res.* 29:355, 1978.

23. Marx, J. L. NMR Research: Analysis of living cells and organisms. *Science* 202:958, 1978.

24. Marx, J. L. NMR researchers embark on new enterprise. *Science* 213:425, 1981.

25. Purcell, E. M. Research in nuclear magnetism. *Science* 118:431, 1953.

26. Ross, B. D., et al. Examination of a case of suspected McArdle's syndrome by ^{31}P nuclear magnetic resonance. *N. Engl. J. Med.* 304:1338, 1981.

Index